COSMIC
HEALTH

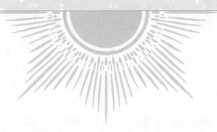

COSMIC HEALTH

UNLOCK YOUR HEALING MAGIC
WITH ASTROLOGY, POSITIVE PSYCHOLOGY,
AND INTEGRATIVE WELLNESS

Jennifer Racioppi

LITTLE, BROWN SPARK
New York   Boston   London

To the Earth, sun, and moon with devoted humility

Contents

Contents

Preface

Before there was Earth, Love, Death, Night, Day, or Light, there was Chaos. Alternately described as a goddess, a "shapeless nothingness," and a "mix of the elements," Chaos gave birth to two children: Erebus, the "unfathomable depth where death dwells," and Night.

Surrounded by a terrifyingly blank and boundless abyss, Night nonetheless placed a wind-born egg into the arms of Erebus. With time, Love burst forth, bringing order and beauty to the bottomless confusion all around.

Love then created Light and, with it, radiant Day. At long last, almighty Earth, also known as Gaia, came into being. A physical container of solid ground, Gaia possessed an equally powerful personality that shifted and changed, interacted and reacted. She was, and remains, almighty yet tender, formidable yet fragile.[1]

She, along with her lineage, lives on all around us, and also inside us. She and her ancestors remain a part of you, me, and all of us.

For too long we have been taught to fear, critique, and tuck away life's chaos, yet in doing so, we forget its immense power to transform us, our health, our lives, as well as the world we live in. While chaos may seem dark and daunting, as the time of Chaos surely was, when we dismiss chaos, we forgo the opportunity to give birth to love, light, radiance, and abundance of every imaginable kind. We unnecessarily dim our own magic. As we dive into this journey, I ask that you, like Chaos herself, resist the temptation to hide and reject your unique brand of chaos and instead embrace it as a sacred invitation into your own cosmic health.

COSMIC
HEALTH

Introduction

Unable to stand, I crawled to the phone and dialed 911. Within minutes, my ninety-seven-pound body was strapped onto a stretcher, and ambulance sirens began echoing through the streets, broadcasting my race to the emergency room. The excruciating abdominal pain that had made me buckle over just minutes earlier had not yet let up. Equally torturous was the anxiety roiling within, consuming what little energy I had left.

It was a hot July day at the Jersey Shore, just six weeks after my eighteenth birthday. While my friends enjoyed the summer sun on the beach, I spent my days, which soon became months, in and out of hospital beds. Weak, depleted, and profoundly unprepared for the journey ahead of me, I drifted through a dark fog of agonizing pain, sleep that failed to relieve my crippling fatigue, and depression that only worsened with wakefulness.

My diagnosis, and its gravity, felt undeniable and terrifying. Aggressive ovarian cancer wreaked havoc on my young, small frame. Or so they told me.

In some ways the diagnosis made sense to me. After years of brutal cramps, chronic depression, and menstrual dysfunction—years during which my doctor repeatedly told me I was a "normal teenager with normal hormonal imbalances"—I felt a small measure of relief from having my intuition validated. As I'd long suspected, I wasn't just a "normal teenager." I'd taken some combination of antidepressants and the pill for years. Yet the extreme suffering caused by my menstrual cycle, which had sometimes forced me to stay home from school, skip the athletics that I loved, and forgo the social chaos of teen life, persisted. My symptoms were anything but typical. That had been clear to me, and now, at long last, it was clear to my doctors too.

And it was cancer, which is to say incredibly daunting. As I underwent an array of procedures and surgeries at various hospitals, I couldn't foresee how volatile, yet enlightening, my health challenges would become. I didn't yet know that after undergoing surgery to remove the bowling-ball-sized tumor from my left ovary, my initial diagnosis would be rescinded. Instead of ovarian cancer, a year later I'd learn I had endometrial cancer.

The cancer was ultimately removed, and with it, my ovaries, uterus, cervix, and fallopian tubes. Not yet twenty years old, I was forced to undergo a radical hysterectomy and face the fact that I would never have biological children. The morning after that surgery, the doctor handed me a yellow, football-shaped pill and told me I'd have to take it every day for the next thirty years. That pill contained the estrogen my body could no longer produce. Despite the synthetic hormone supplementation, the absence of reproductive organs to supply my system with natural estrogen forced my body into menopause—*literally overnight.*

Who at age twenty thinks about the symptoms and implications of menopause? I wasn't remotely prepared for what was to come. Terrified and distressed, I felt completely alone.

Looking back, I now see that I wasn't alone. Even at my lowest of low points, I never was. So many of the women I now work with have their own stories of trauma, disease, heartache, and depression. For years—which sometimes turned into decades—they lived lives punctuated with that same deep soul ache and strong yet muted whispers from inside themselves...*Something is off...This isn't working...Listen to me; please listen.*

Like me, so many women have also had their intuitive knowing repeatedly invalidated by external authority figures. So many of them, like me, have taken themselves and their health to the brink, only to

4

realize that living the body-and-soul nourishing lives they yearn for means ending their reliance on the next quick fix, miracle pill, practice, plan, or belief system. They, too, have faced the fact that our individual and collective pursuits of the one big change — *the* spiritual practice, *the* diet change, and so on — isn't taking us anywhere we want to go.

Instead, we must assume a radical level of responsibility for our health — not just physical but emotional and spiritual too. We must find more authentic and comprehensive ways to heal. Only that kind of all-encompassing, holistic well-being can support the hopes and dreams we're committed to realizing.

For me, the recognition that I needed to take charge of my whole health came after my hysterectomy. In the anxiety-ridden months that followed my final surgery, in the middle of my college years, I moved to the West Coast. There, in the late 1990s, while working as a waitress, I was introduced to a wide array of alternative health and spiritual practices. These mind–body–spirit practices became the foundation of the reclamation of my body, my health, and my life.

One pivotal day at Lake Tahoe, I was fortunate to find my first spiritual mentor, Debbie Lefay, whose petite frame and rhythmic voice belied her powerful yet odd-sounding wisdom.

As she gave me a life-changing tarot reading, I felt a primal tug inside me. We had never met before and social media didn't exist, so she possessed no concrete knowledge of my past. Yet this fairylike creature named my experience so accurately, it almost felt invasive. Did I dare trust her guidance? Would I really experience the healing I desperately needed by claiming a relationship to cyclical living and working with lunar rhythms? I would, according to Debbie.

In those early years, my inner knowing, that fuzzy yet tangible sixth sense we call intuition, often yanked at my science-loving intellect. What was real? What was pure, unhinged woo-woo? What was wisdom passed down through generations, only to be submerged and dismissed in the name of reason, logic, and all things patriarchal?

Debbie taught me that the phases of the moon mirror the menstrual cycle, and that by strategically keying into the moon's cadence, I could connect to the cycle I had lost when I sacrificed my ovaries to survive cancer, a cycle I never knew how to honor due to hormonal dysfunction. It was a fascinating dive into a new realm of understanding that ultimately pulled me in multiple directions.

Then, in 2001, while studying at San Francisco State University, I had the honor of meeting renowned trauma expert Dr. Peter Levine. Inspired by his work, I went into therapy and experienced firsthand the transformative power of healing trauma through his Somatic Experiencing method, which addresses PTSD through a combination of physiology and psychology.

Continuing to integrate moon work into my process, my healing slowly but surely unfolded at the intersection of alternative wellness, nontraditional spirituality, and evidence-based protocols.

Years later, I became certified as a yoga teacher and then as an Ayurvedic nutritionist. I went on to become a certified integrative health coach with a specialty in behavior change at Duke Integrative Medicine. I also studied and apprenticed with leaders in positive psychology and resilience pedagogy—Dr. Maria Sirois and Dr. Tal Ben-Shahar—serving as their teaching assistant.

With each new layer of knowledge and experience, my intellect-based skepticism melted away, and I saw how misguided my assumptions had been. Astrology, spirituality, and integrative medicine don't each exist in a vacuum. They are aligned with, and connected to, science. As my understanding deepened, I discovered that these disciplines are also powerfully connected to one another.

Not only did my studies and ongoing practice improve my physical health, but I also began to experience a deep sense of integration within me. I learned that I am both intuitive and scientific, spiritual as well as brass-tacks—what I've since termed "lunar logic." This union of science and magic allowed me to accept and embrace all of me, and in the process create a life that was aligned with my natural tendencies and the rhythms of the moon that lived inside me. Even now, that growing sense of well-being, while never perfect, is continually reflected back to me through my resilience and my ability to move through difficulty with grace and stamina.

Thanks to this work, over the past decade-plus, I have had the honor of privately coaching hundreds of highly ambitious clients, and supporting many more through my online platform, on their healing journeys as they pursued their life goals without burning out. It brings me profound joy to help them achieve greater health, well-being, and success on their own terms. We do this by honoring the biological and cosmic rhythms that guide their lives, developing a deeper understanding of self through their astrology charts and coaching while integrating simple but powerful mind–body practices. With consistency, they experience the profound sense of confidence and calm that comes from knowing *Whatever comes next, I've got this.*

I'm so excited to share this rich body of work with you. Before we dive in, let's take a quick tour of cosmic health, beginning with an introduction to the core concept.

Introducing Cosmic Health

Cosmic health is at the intersection of cutting-edge research and ancient wisdom, marrying astrology with evidence-based science to create holistic well-being. As a healing path, it honors our individuality, our role in the universe, nature, and the seasonality of life while amplifying emotional, spiritual, and physical health.

Let's break this down a little more.

Astrology studies the correlation between the celestial bodies and events here on Earth. It sheds light on how everyone, and everything, is connected.

By defining the multidimensional significance of our moment of birth through astrology, we gain access to a map that defines our potential. When we then marry that knowledge to the modern evidence-based science of positive psychology and integrative wellness, we can unlock our most natural expression of health, well-being, and happiness.

Cosmic health supports us in building the resilience we need to face life exactly as it is and make it better. It teaches us to live cyclically, how to have a clearer understanding of ourselves, and how to amplify our natural healing capacities.

A Preliminary Note on Health

There is a grave disparity, in the US and in other countries, when it comes to access to healthcare, the ability to practice self-care, the types of stress on marginalized and oppressed peoples, and how different it is for those with economic advantage, especially for those who are white. As a cisgender white woman, I have become keenly aware of how privilege supported my healing.

While this book does not address systemic injustices as an impediment to health, nor is it a book on social justice, it's essential to name systems designed for oppression as a cause of disease and disparity, especially among marginalized populations. Learning to recognize and interrupt oppressive social and economic patterns that keep society unwell is a part of our cosmic health.

Cosmic health is about gaining the tools we need to have more resilience so we can rewire our internal systems and walk a path to more wellness and well-being, despite the challenges we face. Being well in a society designed to keep us sick is revolutionary.

Similarly, disrupting definitions of health remains paramount too.

So many of us live with chronic illnesses that will likely never be cured, myself included. Whatever Western medicine may have told us, let me say this:

We absolutely can achieve optimal wellness while living with illness. The National Wellness Institute defines wellness as a "self-directed and evolving process" that's "multidimensional and holistic...Wellness is positive and affirming."[1] Achieving wellness doesn't require perfection. It isn't just resolving specific symptoms. It is striving to create resilient lives, no matter the obstacles. We can stay faithful to our wellness journey, even in the face of incurable diseases.

And we can embrace nonconventional spirituality on the healing journey without denying evidence-based science or our intellects. We can also see illness for the opportunity it often offers us: to make soul-directed changes that bring us into deeper congruency with who we really are so we can rise.

How to Use This Book

The spirit that resides in your body, the one that animates all of life, has an uncanny ability to work its miracles, no matter the obstacles you face. You come to this book with your own life experiences and cultural history, but we all share one thing: we are cosmic beings. I hope that as you read this book you will take what applies to you and use it to mobilize your healing magic.

In the chapters that follow, you'll find my own stories and stories from the ambitious clients I coach, like Isobel, Carina, Claire, Mari, and many more. While they all use the pronouns she/her, and this book is for anyone who identifies as a woman, cosmic health's principles can be adapted to apply to nonbinary people and men.

Throughout the book, I've incorporated stories of powerful mythological archetypes, which I use as guiding lights in my own life and in my teaching. They provide such valuable role models of what it means to embody the full range of our multifaceted nature—to be loving and nurturing yet fierce and determined too.

In the book, you'll also find journaling prompts and mantras to help you integrate what you've learned and attune your inner cosmos to the outer cosmos. I've included rituals too—some action-oriented, others more reflective—to help you implement your cosmic health insights in a practical, accessible way.

You can read this book from beginning to end or immerse yourself in a chapter that calls to you. A fundamental tenet of cosmic health is the idea that health is not a one-and-done mastery but a continuous journey. Remember, the healing process is just that, a process. Come back to each section as often as you need.

In my work and in this book, I use astrology as a tool for self-discovery and self-development, not to predict the future or diagnose disease. Instead, I use astrology as a way to help uncover a person's strengths and weaknesses so that person can consciously harness their own healing, grow their resilience, and self-actualize.

My goal in writing this book is to marry key concepts from astrology with correlative research and concepts from positive psychology and integrative wellness, but please note this is not exhaustive or definitive. Nor is this a training in astrology, or the only astrology book you'll ever need. I will introduce you to some of the key components of the natal chart, but this book is not intended to teach you how to interpret your chart.

In part I of the book, you'll explore the five principles of cosmic health as well as the connection between astrology and health. By the end of this section you'll be prepped with the mindset and tools to start exploring your health in a whole new way.

In part II, you'll be introduced to cyclical living. At this point you will begin to put your new understanding into practice and experience the rhythmicity of living in sync with solar and lunar cycles.

In part III, you'll explore the core components of your astro-individuality: your sun, moon, and rising signs. Understanding these components will help you digest your core astrological makeup. We'll break down these key parts of your natal chart — your astrological blue-print at birth — to grasp how the cosmos informs your particular needs and conspires to make you uniquely awesome. (We will take a look at these components of your astrology, as well as other celestial influences, through the signs but not through the houses. Communicating the full significance of the houses, especially as they pertain to your personal chart, is a huge undertaking and not one I can sufficiently address in this book.)

Given the pivotal role that emotions play in mind–body science and holistic health, we'll begin by looking at your natal moon sign, which has a substantial influence on your deeper emotional needs and well-being. We'll also identify specific rituals to help you amplify your energy, gain more focus, and care for your overall well-being through thick and thin.

In part IV, the heart of the book, you'll explore the remaining celestial bodies—Mercury, Venus, Mars, Jupiter, Saturn, Chiron, Uranus, Neptune, and Pluto—and look at how they affect you, your life, and the new rhythm you're beginning to implement and benefit from.[2]

By this point in the process, you'll have full and unfettered access to what I refer to as your superpowers—the blend of traits and tendencies that makes you uniquely and amazingly *you*. This is where your personal brand of cosmic health lives. Understand, this isn't a fairy dust type of magic but a very real-world kind of awesomeness that you will learn to harness in service of your health and your life.

Many of my clients have used this approach to achieve an all-encompassing sense of health and well-being while simultaneously creating purpose-driven careers, more supportive and intimate relationships, and a more connected homelife. Many have also begun to practice seasonal and intuitive eating, create new relationships with their bodies and movement, and gain confidence, not just in their physical selves but in deeply rooted feelings of connection, meaning, and purpose. They have embraced a self-directed journey of emotional well-being and spiritual alignment, and cultivated their resilience as a path to change.

Regardless of the challenges you may be facing, this book will show you how to unlock the fierce well-being you've yearned for. I can't wait to get started, so that you, too, can join the thousands who have used this body of work to transform their lives into fulfilling and multidimensional reflections of their *cosmic health*.

Part I

FIRE

Understanding Cosmic Health

If one opens up chaos, magic also arises.
—C. G. JUNG, FROM *THE RED BOOK*

CHAPTER 1

The Five Principles of Cosmic Health

My journey, like those of so many of my clients, and perhaps also like yours, began with crisis and chaos. Consumed by misery and fear, and near hopelessness, I was scared that I'd lost not just my way but also my chance at health and happiness. It is a deeply disheartening place to begin. From that place we fumble, stumble, and fall—as we are meant to. Yet immersed in that darkest of darkness, we, like the goddess Chaos, are destined to find Love and Light.

Know this: this book is not your typical health book. It guides you in figuring out how to view your own chaos as a sacred door into your deeper desires for success, however you define it, and self-realization. While its impact is profound, it does not rush in to "fix" anything or anyone.

As dispiriting as your chaos may now seem, throughout this journey you can and will use it to facilitate many internal and external transformations.

We'll focus first on the five core components, or principles, of cosmic health:

Principle 1: Live cyclically.
Principle 2: Build resilience, a key to health.

Principle 3: Know thyself… It is a never-ending adventure.
Principle 4: Embrace the paradox of "both/and."
Principle 5: Unlock your healing magic.

Before we explore these principles in depth, we need to bust some of the popular myths about both the cosmic and our health. Having that solid grounding will enable you—like it has so many others we'll meet in the coming pages—to navigate the ebbs and flows of life in ways that feel supportive and empowering.

Kosmos and the Cosmic

My interpretation of "cosmic" integrates all iterations of the word, from the ancient *kosmos* to the present-day "cosmos."

In ancient Greek, *kosmos* meant "beautiful order"[1]—a well-assembled whole that beautifies life. Today, we use the word "cosmos" to describe the universe as a literal collection of stars, planets, and the moon—that vast, awe-inspiring image we see in the night sky. To some, the cosmos is also a magical, mystical realm described in reverential spiritual terms.

When I talk about the cosmos, I mean "cosmic" to refer to *all* the pieces of your health and wellness: mental, spiritual, emotional, and physical. Realizing your cosmic health means assembling the different parts of yourself and your well-being to create your own "beautiful order." By integrating astrology into these aspects of your life, you gain access to the wisdom and guidance of the cosmos as we know it today, creating a powerful relationship with the rhythm and flow of the universe.

A Fresh Perspective on Health

Now that we've established the meaning of "cosmic" as it pertains to cosmic health, let's look at "health."

Western medicine typically defines health as the absence of disease.

As a cancer survivor, a health practitioner, and someone who manages life while living with a chronic illness, I find that definition limiting and unfairly exclusive. According to that definition, I and many of my friends, clients, and family are not, and can never be, healthy.

I have great respect and appreciation for Western medicine, which—let's be honest—played a huge role in my surviving cancer. However, when it comes to defining "health," I opt for a less traditional and more inclusive interpretation. Rather than define health by what it's not—disease—I see health as a way of both being and becoming. It's a multidimensional awareness that nurtures your physical existence, your spiritual and creative prowess, your intellectual desires, and, last but certainly not least, your emotional health.

Cosmic health embraces imperfection, can endure setbacks, and can even coexist with disease. It grants you the capacity to evolve in highly personalized ways, adapting to life's ups and downs while living a full and thriving life.

The cosmic health I want for you, the state of being and becoming I will lead you toward in this book, will allow you to cultivate compassion for yourself and others while living a life drenched in meaning and beauty. That meaning and beauty won't come from the superficial satisfaction of achievements and appearances. Instead, it will stem from cultivating the self-awareness that's essential to self-actualizing at the highest level.

This may not sound like any definition of health you've heard before. That's because we've been sold so many myths about health and what it means to be healthy, including:

- Being healthy means being perfect: attaining the perfect BMI, following an eating plan perfectly for the rest of your life, having a perfectly consistent exercise regimen, and being perfectly free from disease.
- Being healthy means achieving an unfaltering and unfluctuating life balance.

- Being healthy means having a body that looks a certain way.
- Being healthy means living stress-free.
- Being healthy takes hard work, discipline, and sacrifice. To be healthy, we have to experience *less* pleasure and have *less* fun.

These cultural beliefs around health often lead us away from true health and wellness. Unwilling to forgo pleasure, we may abandon the pursuit of vibrant health. Or, obsessed with becoming *perfectly* healthy, we go all in and rely on deprivation and strict routines that steal the joy and connection that would enhance, rather than detract from, our health. Others among us may yo-yo, bounding from one extreme (deprivation and rigidity) to another (total indulgence) and back again.

Cultivating a Healthier Relationship with Health

In order to achieve cosmic health, we first need to repair and broaden our relationship with health itself. Let's take a look at some myths about health and start adopting more empowering beliefs around what it means to be healthy.

MYTH: *Balance is essential to healthy living.*

A world-renowned musician. A successful entrepreneur. A corporate executive, wife, and mom. All of these people are clients of mine who, like you, have been taught that life balance is one of the holy grails of healthful living. Truth be told, these clients actually want to unleash their own genius. They want to manage their energy, not their time, and, in so doing, commune with their mysticism to make a major difference in the world—even when that means temporarily sacrificing balance.

We yearn for self-actualization. We yearn to become a better version of ourselves as thoroughly and as often as we can. We yearn to feel fulfilled and connected, successful and thriving. We yearn to serve the greater good. We want a lot, and we're prepared to go for all of it.

Just like Earth and the moon, life oscillates. It *changes*, evolving from one season to the next. We, too, naturally cycle through beginnings, periods of culmination, and then periods that wane. Because of this, we move from order to chaos and back to order again. Being able to flex alongside this ever-changing rhythm, again and again, is the true manifestation of health. To do that we have to first accept that rhythmic adaptation—not balance—is what will support our ability to have a greater impact. It's also what best supports our cosmic health.

MYTH: *Optimal health is an exclusively physical state of being.*

Health isn't an appearance. Nor is it defined by the absence of disease, being an "ideal" size, or having the "perfect" spiritual practice. Health depends as much on our emotional well-being—including our ability to digest uncertainty and challenge—as it does on having a functional physical body.

When we meet emotions with curiosity, humility, and a willingness to understand them within the contexts of past and present, including the cosmic conditions at our birth and at present, we can move into and through them. This willingness to feel our emotions can't just extend to positive emotions. It also must encompass gnarly emotions like rage, fear, shame, and sadness, all of which are part of the human experience.

By incorporating emotional well-being into our search for health, we can heal the many different, interconnected parts of ourselves. One client of mine experienced this kind of healing when she decided to end a long-term relationship. Although she was scared of being alone and felt overwhelmed by her emotions, with time, space, and support, she learned to feel her feelings. She also realized that experiencing her full range of emotions made her healthier and more resilient.

MYTH: *Your health should be as close to perfect as possible.*

We live in a time of rapid healthcare innovation and evolution, so much so that we've come to believe that everything can and must be cured. Too often we're sold on the idea that peak health is a state we can and should reach and maintain forever. This just isn't true. Nor is it possible. I live with a chronic illness and continue to thrive despite my health challenges, and you can too.

Being healthy means constantly changing, growing, and becoming. We've been taught to be wary of transitional spaces yet, as master life coach and bestselling author Nancy Levin says, we must "honor the space between no longer and not yet." Doing so is how we transform into better, more authentic versions of ourselves.

"Imperfect" is healthy, beautiful, and where we need to place our long-term focus.

MYTH: *Stress is bad for our health.*

For too long we've demonized stress when, in fact, stress and self-actualization often go hand in hand. Think about the last time you experienced growth in your life, like when you had to perform a new task, make a big move, or even get married. All of these life-affirming activities come with significant stress.

Stress accompanies growth. Avoiding stress can keep us from evolving, which is counterproductive to health. Instead, our focus needs to be on understanding and managing stress. This includes learning how to lean into stress and grow stronger, smarter, more creative, and more fulfilled as a result.

In order to reap the powerful rewards that navigating stress can deliver, we must prioritize replenishment as much as we do productivity. This means eating for nourishment, sleeping for energy, living for joy, de-escalating stress, finding rewarding purpose in our work, and developing life-giving intimacy with those we love.

This cycle of depletion and replenishment happens continuously in the body. Every day fifty to seventy billion cells in the human body die, and in that same period, it creates an equivalent number of new cells. Similarly, to build muscle we first have to inflict muscle damage by lifting weights or doing strenuous cardio. To prevent long-term injury, we then have to give our muscles time to recover.

On emotional and spiritual levels, we also experience this depletion-replenishment cycle. Depletion, which might appear as dips in energy, lack of motivation, disappointment, challenges, or chaos, is a reality of life. Being healthy means being able to face life as it is, rather than as it "should" be, while simultaneously moving in the direction we choose. In that process, we must also take breaks and recharge our emotional and spiritual "batteries."

On every level, our health is intimately connected to our ability to rise to the challenges we face and then recover from those energy expenditures.

MYTH: *Being healthy is hard work.*

We've been sold on achieving extreme health—"perfect" health—and we've continually fallen short of meeting these impossible expectations. Constantly striving for perfection and chasing health contribute to burnout, depletion, and feelings of shame. Being healthy is an enjoyable, natural state, especially when we attune to a more cyclical way of living. We'll begin to look at that next.

The Core Principles of Cosmic Health

Now that we've busted some of the myths about health and the cosmos, let's bring these concepts together into a clear picture of what cosmic health means for you. The five principles mentioned earlier and laid out in this section are ones we'll come back to again and again. They're also skills you'll develop as you progress through this book. Think of them as guardrails to keep you in the cosmic health lane.

PRINCIPLE 1: *Live cyclically.*

The sun rises and sets. The moon waxes and wanes. We live on a planet that rotates on its axis, alternating between day, an extended period of light, and night, a roughly equivalent period of darkness. These are small examples of how the cosmos operates cyclically.

Our bodies also act and react cyclically. The human body (plants and animals too) biologically responds to fluctuations of light and dark. Most cells and tissues in the body run on molecular "clocks" that operate most effectively when they synchronize with the external light–dark cycle they mirror.

For example, the circadian rhythm, which is the twenty-four-hour cycle that regulates our sleep and waking times, works best when it syncs with the cycle of night and day.

Like an operator controlling a phone bank, this rhythm supports brain function, first, by reporting to the hypothalamus gland, a tiny portion of the brain that is roughly the size of an almond. The hypothalamus works in concert with the pituitary gland to fire up the adrenals, which create the hormone cortisol in the morning, alerting us to rise, followed by melatonin at night, making us feel sleepy. This major neuroendocrine relationship, known as the HPA axis, controls our autonomic nervous system and sets the stage for healthy hormone function during each part of the twenty-four-hour cycle. This diurnal/nocturnal, or day and night, hormonal oscillation acts as a foundation for all cognitive functioning. As a result, by living in alignment with the natural cycle of light and dark dictated by Earth's daily rotation and yearly revolution around the sun, we allow our bodies to function better.

When we live out of sync with the natural cycles of light—for example, by exposing ourselves to too much artificial light at night or by failing to sleep—this natural internal clock is disrupted. The hypothalamus fails to do its job and the hormonal symphony it creates doesn't synchronize. Metabolic function, mood, and cognition are all compromised, performance suffers, and the mood-boosting chemical serotonin dips too low. This inevitably drives us to push ourselves harder, which only causes us to slip further into the abyss of feeling crappy. While all this happens, our immune system weakens, which makes us more vulnerable to health challenges.

Living out of sync with solar and cosmic cycles comes at a great cost, yet it's an all too common scenario in a modern society that perpetually overrides these natural rhythms. Our calendars and schedules suggest that these essential cycles don't matter. We banish darkness with artificial light and tech devices. We work and rest according to a clock, not the rising and setting of the sun. While I am not suggesting we forgo electricity and only sleep and wake with the sun, I am pointing out the value of honoring our biological rhythms.

The practice of setting up your environment to support your circadian rhythm, known as circadian entrainment, helps to optimize your body's process of living rhythmically. Returning to a life that's more in sync with circadian and cosmic rhythms is an important step toward mental, emotional, and physical well-being. Small, simple practices, like shutting down digital devices at a certain hour each night, can help us achieve this.

This circadian rhythm is a powerful tonic but not the only rhythm that affects us. Two other rhythms that influence us are "ultradian" and "infradian." An ultradian rhythm is a rhythm shorter than twenty-four hours, often repeating multiple times through the day. The most common one is the basic rest-activity cycle, or BRAC. This cycle happens at 80-to-20-minute intervals and influences our energy and focus and our REM vs. non-REM sleep cycles. Infradian rhythms occur in longer segments. For example, the monthly menstrual cycle runs on an infradian rhythm, mirroring the circalunar rhythm of the moon. The body's biological response to the seasons is also an infradian rhythm, known as the circannual rhythm.

We don't have to dissect or even understand every one of the cycles we encounter, but we do need to recognize that life is a rhythm inside a rhythm inside a rhythm. We're constantly in a dance with our internal beat and the beats of the universe and planets.

Living cyclically, aligned with the cycles of the sun and moon, is the most natural thing you'll ever do. *It's what you are physically, mentally, and emotionally designed to do.* Your body was built to work according to these cycles. The trick is to stop expending valuable time and energy fighting these rhythms and, instead, concede to them—because they guide so much of our biology. When we live in sync with them, everything becomes easier.

PRINCIPLE 2: *Build resilience, a key to health.*

In order to manage the ever-changing nature of our lives and health, we must be able to navigate the space between what is and what will be. We need to be able to endure, and leverage, chaos. That requires an ever-growing reserve of resilience.

Resilience is the capacity to face and adapt to change and also recover from challenges. It is a concept and way of being that applies to individuals, groups of people, and communities. With resilience, we can not only bounce back from disaster, disappointment, and setbacks but also grow stronger because of them. In doing so, we develop a sense of mastery in our lives.

While its benefits are widely appreciated, resilience itself is often misunderstood. Resilience doesn't mean that we forgo grief or avoid or suppress the pain we feel at turbulent times in our lives. Nor is resilience a "no pain, no gain" mentality, or about having a "stiff upper lip," or persevering at any cost.

To become truly resilient, it's critical that we sensitize ourselves to our emotions and, when necessary, allow ourselves to process the full force of their range. From a health standpoint, repressing, suppressing, or denying emotions can manifest as physical symptoms, encompassing everything from chronic pain to insomnia, headaches, weight fluctuations, hormonal imbalances, and more—all of which can contribute to disease.

Developing resilience means understanding our emotions and feeling them *while also* moving our lives forward. Maintaining our resilience, and the resilience of our communities, requires our humanity. It's relational work. To become truly resilient, we must nurture and honor our sensitivity, not push it aside.

COMMON TRAITS OF RESILIENT PEOPLE

To give you a more complete understanding of what resilience looks like in individuals, here are common traits that resilient people often share:

They maintain meaningful relationships and a strong network of social support.

Dr. Maria Sirois, my positive psychology mentor whose teachings influenced my thinking on resilience, taught me the power of cultivating a choir over a posse. Rather than relying on a posse, or a group of people to *fit in with,* we instead need a choir, a group to which *we truly belong.* A choir supports us during tough times as well as our best moments. Even when we don't have a choir of people, we can build a choir within ourselves through self-care, bonding with a beloved animal, or connecting to artists, musicians, or poets whose work resonates with us deeply. Nature can be a part of our choir too. Having support that nourishes us in our times of both difficulty and happiness aids our thriving.

They see the world through rose-colored realism.

While the large-scale popularity of positive psychology has proven powerful and advantageous in many ways, the true meaning and message of positive psychology has also been distorted into positive mythology. In fact, optimism at any cost is neither productive nor supportive. Unbridled, ungrounded optimism more often prevents us from initiating the changes that ultimately boost our resilience.

In truth, positive thoughts alone cannot deliver the outcomes we desire. However, optimism that's accompanied by a sense of realism, which I call "rose-colored realism," is about being a realist *and* a consummate benefit finder: someone who can find the benefit in, and even discern the meaning of, the stresses of life.

They invest in trust, faith, and gratitude.

When we live in sync with our internal and external rhythms, we can cultivate a deeper trust in them. Rooted in this trust, we can embrace the fact that each period of waning, however long or trying, will be followed by a period of waxing—that each dip will be met with a subsequent rise. Knowing this, we can cultivate gratitude amidst the ebb and flow of life. Faith, which I'm using here in a nontraditional, nondenominational sense, connects us to awe, wonder, compassion, and gratitude. It also gives us the capacity to forgive, allowing us to cultivate a more profound sense of belonging and connection within our families and communities. When we invest in trust and faith—in ourselves, the universe, and the rhythms of our lives—we can see, believe in, and be grateful for the basic goodness of the universe. Throughout this book, we'll explore spirituality from this lens of cultivating trust and faith, both as a personal experience and as a broader cosmic one.

They embrace their innate creativity—and make sure to laugh in the process.

When we continually practice creative thinking, options and answers to even the most challenging situations often become apparent. The more we allow ourselves to laugh and feel joy, the easier and more naturally our creativity flows. Together, creativity and laughter empower us to bounce back from challenges while also discovering new and innovative solutions.

They live with grit.

The more aligned we become with our truth and purpose, the more likely we are to go for our big dreams. That inevitably increases the stress and challenges we face. By developing grit—which Angela Duckworth, the *New York Times*–bestselling author of *Grit,* defines as a "combination of perseverance and passion"—we become better able to handle what comes our way with unrelenting tenacity. Her book is brilliantly written, and I particularly like how she describes grit in the FAQ section of her website. "Grit is about having what some researchers call an 'ultimate concern' — a goal you care about so much that it organizes and gives meaning to almost everything you do. And grit is holding steadfast to that goal. Even when you fall down. Even when you screw up. Even when progress toward that goal is halting or slow. Talent and luck matter to success. But talent and luck are no guarantee of grit. And in the very long run, I think grit may matter at least as much, if not more."[2]

When we fail or are disappointed by outcomes that don't meet expectations, we try again or find a new solution. That's grit. By developing grit, we become better able to get back up after setbacks. Grit requires uncompromising commitment.

PRINCIPLE 3: *Know thyself...It is a never-ending adventure.*

Who you were yesterday isn't necessarily who you are today, and who you are today may not be who you are next week. Like the cosmos, you are constantly changing. You will never be "finished." When you embrace growth and change as fundamental building blocks of health, you give yourself ample and ongoing permission to transform. Your identity is constantly adapting, which also means that you're forever in the process of getting to know yourself.

That continual process of getting to know yourself is essential to creating cosmic health.

By applying this evolutionary mindset to the self-awareness journey, we become more flexible and willing to make new and different choices that reflect and support our most radiant health. This is a form of mindful living, in which we stay rooted in the present and notice and respond to what the body, mind, and soul need at any given point in time.

Rather than pursuing one-size-fits-all health trends, we *can* slow down, listen, and tailor our health and self-care to meet our *individual* needs and desires. Instead of making decisions to meet other people's expectations or demands, we can be guided by a strong, clear sense of self-knowing and purpose. We're in a never-ending dance between knowing and becoming, and navigating this requires adaptability and abundant, unrelenting self-acceptance.

By integrating astrology into the process, we can better understand that predetermined aspects of life do not rob us of our power or agency. We can adapt and evolve. By continually getting to know ourselves, we can discern which behaviors, actions, and patterns best serve us at different times. Our unique relationship to Earth, the sun, the moon, and the other planets, seen through the lens of astrology, provides a map of our becoming.

PRINCIPLE 4: *Embrace the paradox of "both/and."*

Cosmic health embraces what Jim Collins, author of *Built to Last*, calls the "genius of the and" over "the tyranny of the or."[3] Health isn't either/or; it's both/and. The rational and the unquantifiable *can* coexist.

You can take care of your emotional well-being and mind–body health *and* treat illness with the best of what Western medicine has to offer.

You can have a strong sense of individual identity *and* experience the benefits of understanding collective meaning.

You can accept that you have behavioral predispositions predicated by an astrology chart *and* work on how you express those traits.

You can live in awe, marveling at the mystery of the universe and your body, *and* still love science.

You can honor ancient wisdom (astrology) *and* modern science (positive psychology, integrative wellness, and more).

When it comes to your wellness journey and health goals, you can take care of who you are now *and* still hold a strong vision for who you want to be in the future. It's not a mutually exclusive journey. You can see illness, stress, and chaos as directives for what needs to change without negating or ignoring the intensity they unleash.

Finding the "and" applies to all aspects of our lives.

We are finite *and* expansive. We are distinct individuals *and* parcels of the same cosmos.

We can grieve *and* feel happy. We can have a chronic illness *and* be healthy. We can experience moments of extreme stress *and* evolve toward our highest good.

We can search for health *and* still be filled with joy. We can live with a wound that never totally heals *and* still self-actualize.

We can be well-adjusted humans with high-functioning lives *and* still experience hardship, melancholy, anger, and pain.

We can be both scientific *and* magical. We can be realists *and* full of hope too.

Cosmic health is a strong but graceful methodology that embodies sensitivity while having an impact. It produces very real results but in ways that feel gentle *and* powerful too.

PRINCIPLE 5: *Unlock your healing magic.*

As women, we've long been shamed out of owning our power, coerced into being conciliatory, accommodating, and nurturing. While those attributes may be part of who we are, we are also the embodiment of both/and. Our loving-kindness exists in alignment with the immense, often underrealized potency that bubbles deep inside us. Using astrology, positive psychology, and integrative wellness to bolster our cosmic health, we simultaneously unlock our sovereignty as well as the possibility inherent within us and in the natural world around us.

Historically, healing magic was deemed "witchery," brushed off as nonsensical madness or, at its most extreme, viewed as a crime punishable by death. For the "crime" of claiming their knowledge and using the healing powers of nature, thousands of women were tortured and sacrificed. However ancient that history may seem, our strength and the zest it triggers are still continually invalidated and maligned. It's not surprising — by reclaiming our healing magic, we reclaim our power, and by reclaiming our power, we awaken ferocity inside us. Both scenarios are unacceptable in a patriarchal society.

The dominant social institutions of centuries past (and even today) feared the implications of this sort of self-possession. How could they control a population that subscribed to such personal empowerment? So they cast a disdainful shadow on it, labeling anything subversive as malefic witchery, as a means of oppression.

Our modern-day understanding—and mobilization—of alchemy is very much rooted in its history as a persecuted practice.[4] Historically, people have turned to it in times they have felt the most powerless: when they were oppressed and disenfranchised by society, when their environment— even their own bodies—felt completely out of their own control. Today still, in a society wrought with discrimination based on gender, race, body size, sexual preference, religion, ability, and more, our sacred connection to nature provides a path to reclaiming personal agency and health.

As we embark on this journey, let's first get clear about what healing magic is.

Healing is a therapeutic process of tending to pain. It's the act of restoring health and vitality where wounding has occurred. The goal of healing is renewal, restoration, and improvement. Magic is an act of creation through intention and will, in communion with forces inside ourselves and in the natural world.

Healing magic amplifies our ability to withstand and recover from pain. It's a sacred medicine that helps unlock greater strength and capacity within. It honors our cyclical nature and amplifies our ability to flourish, no matter the circumstances at hand.

Our self-ownership and connection to the cosmos are intrinsic to our healing magic; each necessitates the other. By aligning with the cosmos and nature, we develop the capacity to stay with our healing process even when it feels elusive. Healing, after all, is cyclical, not always progressive. Still, through unearthing our sacred desires, we amplify our ability to, potentially, bend our experience of reality into a desired form.

Healing magic is inside us and all around us, and accessing it supports our transmutation of chaos into cosmic order.

Healing magic unfolds when seemingly disparate parts of our lives click in previously unimaginable ways. It graces us in the form of abundance — in love, work, play, friendship, laughter, vitality, and more.

Healing magic shows up as synchronicity that occurs *despite* the limits of time and space. It appears as the seemingly nonsensical, made manifest. It happens in little ways and big ones.

To reclaim our healing magic, we merely have to open ourselves to it, be willing to see our chaos as a threshold to change, and share our healing magic with a universe that yearns to conjure with us and alongside us. This is what we will do in this book, as we conjure *cosmic health*.

CHAPTER 2

Astrology and Health

I'd never thought of myself as a grounded person. I certainly didn't feel grounded when I first began working with Debra Silverman, a psychotherapist who integrates astrology into her practice. Up until that point in my life, I'd considered myself to be flighty, as in, the polar opposite of grounded.

While that so-called flighty mutable air energy was reflected in my Gemini sun, Libra rising, and Gemini Mercury, those placements were only one part of my cosmic map. With my natal moon, Saturn, and north node all in Virgo, I also had a lot of grounded (earth) energy. When you couple that with a Venus and Mars conjunction in fixed earth Taurus, as Debra showed me, the highest-ranking element in my chart is earth, not air. (If this is too much astrological detail, don't worry. By the end of the book, it will make more sense.)

This earth influence in my chart was a revelation for me. I didn't need to change who I was; I simply had to continue to embrace my healing journey and learn how to align with that grounded part of myself.

As I continued working with Debra, I began connecting to my earthiness and cultivating other aspects of my astrological chart. The emotional and mindset shifts that resulted prompted me to naturally make important changes that had very real and positive impacts on my health.

In this way and many others, integrating astrology into my health and wellness journey changed my life—and since then, it has also changed the lives and health of my clients. Those transformations began with understanding what I now call the "cosmic curriculum." We'll discuss that shortly, but first let's look at how astrology ties to health.

Astrology as a Health Tool

The influence of astrology on Jung's thinking was penetrating and profound, as was his own influence on modern astrologers.

—LIZ GREENE, FROM *JUNG'S STUDIES IN ASTROLOGY*

Some of the greatest scientists and thinkers throughout history have held faithfully to the study of astrology for guidance on health and wellness. Carl Jung, the Swiss psychologist who founded analytical psychology and was arguably one of the most influential thinkers of the twentieth century, utilized astrology both personally and professionally as he developed analytical psychology. He embraced the paradox of the both/and.[1] Jung demonstrated what it means to be both a mystic and a scholar. As a medical doctor and an empiricist, he held the laboratorial rigor of traditional science in high esteem yet continued to use astrology in his practice even though he never could definitively explain how astrology works.[2]

I, like so many of my colleagues, took to astrology for the same reason that Jung continued to use it: it works really well. Unlike the next juice or exercise craze, the rhythm of Earth's motions in relationship to the sun, and the cyclical patterns of the moon, will always influence our wellness states, whether we are paying attention to them or not.

Everything Is Connected

As above, so below. As within, so without. As the universe,
so the soul.

—Hermes Trismegistus

Inherent in Jung's and other scholars' understanding of astrology, and indeed inherent in astrology itself, is the underlying assumption that all things and people are interconnected.

This idea isn't even sort of new. It dates back to the ancient Stoic concept of "cosmic sympathy," also known as "universal sympathy." Cosmic sympathy suggests that all beings on Earth are inextricably linked to one another and the heavens through an organic interrelation that unifies them in an interdependent field. From this view, nothing in the universe can function independently, and everything remains intricately linked. This idea leans into the concept of anima mundi, or "world soul," which Plato adhered to. It means that not only is everything interconnected and interrelated but everything also shares a soul or intelligence.[3]

HOW YOU ARE CONNECTED
TO THE STARS

You are stardust. Yes, you.

[M]ost of the material that we're made of comes out of dying stars, or stars that died in explosions. And those stellar explosions continue. We have stuff in us as old as the universe, and then some stuff that landed here maybe only a hundred years ago. And all of that mixes in our bodies.[4]

According to astrophysicist Karel Schrijver, coauthor of *Living with the Stars: How the Human Body Is Connected to the Life Cycles* of the Earth, the Planets, and the Stars, our bodies are actually and literally made of stardust.

Your body is connected to the same organic material that falls from the sky after a star burns out, and so is the food you eat, the water you drink, and the planet you live on. All of the resources you absorb daily to survive are connected to the greater cosmic forces. Your existence, intricately linked to everything else in existence, embodies the totality of the universe.

How This Interconnectedness Affects Health

With this understanding that we're interconnected—all people and all things—the question becomes, how does this connectedness manifest in our health and our lives?

The answer can be summed up in one word: cycles.

The universe adheres to cycles. Every cycle is a process of transformation with a beginning, middle, and end. From comets in the sky to hormones in the body, aspects of the body and our world follow periods of waxing and waning, depletion and regeneration. All of these cycles co-occur, often in contradiction with one another.

Astrology puts these interconnected elements and their movements into context, which helps us find meaning and create more profound coherence within ourselves and our lives. This coherence supports us in many ways. It helps us make sense of our existence, which has the power to amplify our health and well-being. This will ensure that we have a solid "why" when it comes to taking action and making changes on behalf of our health. It also helps us better understand the timing of the natural world and universe, so we can sync our health practices to the cycles that govern our biology and our lives.

By integrating astrology into how you manage your health and your life, you'll be able to embrace the rising and falling of your body's natural rhythms, maximizing the regeneration process while offsetting the impacts of the degeneration process too. In its most quitescence, astrology maps the very same cycles that the biological rhythms of our body mirror. The different lunar and solar cycles and how they affect you will be dissected in chapters 3 and 4, but for now, keep in mind that cycles play an important role in astrology and your cosmic health.

The Cosmic Curriculum

I was in my mid-twenties when I began working with Debra Silverman. While I'd survived cancer and my hysterectomy, and recovered from depression and debilitating panic attacks, my health and well-being were still less than ideal. None of my symptoms were debilitating or critical, but I knew I needed to take them seriously. I experienced intense heart palpitations that left me frightened and panicked. Digestion issues caused me to feel tired and drained. I also found myself at a crossroads with my professional life, uncertain of my relationship with my partner, and ready to make significant changes.

Debra pointed out several different ways my personal astrology might be affecting my health and lifestyle choices. She highlighted the lack of water energy in my chart, which could make me excessively rigid and resistant to feeling my emotions. With my natal moon in Virgo, she noted, I was more vulnerable to digestive issues. She helped me understand my natal chart and my cosmic curriculum.

Each one of us has a cosmic curriculum, which is the unique and specific trajectory of growth created by the astrological placements that were in play at our moment of birth. Embedded in this curriculum are, of course, lessons that we each need to learn, putting our struggles into a constructive context.

When we view struggles as part of our cosmic curriculum, we're less prone to feeling cosmically rejected or betrayed. Tending to our health becomes productive instead of futile and punitive. In this frame of mind, we can see our struggles as cosmic invitations to achieve growth that's so profound it's only attainable by navigating sizable challenges. That perspective enables us to stay present and open, able to find meaning in the seemingly random chaos of life. By leveraging our problems, we also build resilience for our specific life path and develop the grit to stay focused on our most heartfelt goals and desires, no matter what.

As a typical Gemini, afraid to miss out on opportunities and fun, I often felt like I had to say yes to everything. As a result, I was perpetually overextended. Debra asked me to challenge this pattern and instead commit to living in sync with the rhythms that guided my life. This meant no more working or socializing well past midnight. It also meant loosening my schedule by leaning into my seemingly irrational yearnings to exercise at midday. Instead of sticking to a strict, unforgiving workday schedule, I experimented even more with managing my energy, not my time, which pushed me to prioritize midday movement. As a Libra rising, doing so caused me to deal with my fear of not being liked by others; I mean, going against the grain of standard workday practices rattled every people-pleasing bone in my body. Learning how to undo the "dis-ease to please" (a common Libra-rising trait) and take care of myself felt like liberation.

To address my Virgo-influenced digestion issues, I discovered my gluten allergy. As I adjusted my eating accordingly, I also tackled another underlying factor affecting my digestion and the cause of my heart palpitations: the synthetic estrogen hormonal supplement I'd taken for years. Eager to feel better, I decided to transition to a biodynamic equivalent.

Thanks in part to my having entered menopause years prior, that transition proved far more challenging than I'd imagined. As soon as I went off the synthetic estrogen, my physical body and my emotions went into a tailspin that left me feeling powerless and afraid. It had me crying the ugly-cry, questioning my sanity and my commitment to change. But I stayed the course because I viewed those challenges as part of my cosmic curriculum. Ultimately, that transition put me on a much safer trajectory with my hormone replacement therapy. Thankfully, I haven't had a heart palpitation since.

By helping me to get a handle on my cosmic curriculum, astrology enabled me to infuse purpose and meaning into the rough patches of my healing journey. Rather than feeling like prolonged exercises of infinite torture and punishment, my struggles began to look and feel like robust gateways to accelerated growth, which is what they became.

The Cosmic Curriculum and Spiritual/ Creative Transformation

Sara, a corporate executive, was seeking a life overhaul when she came to me for coaching. As a white woman who had grown up in a Southern patriarchal family, she had long seen her gender and her body as weaknesses, especially since she had experienced sexual abuse in her childhood. Despite the fact that she loved being a woman, she wrestled with the inherent vulnerability she felt in having a female body. Because of this, she identified with the aggressive, whatever-it-takes side of her Aries personality. However, she had recently had a gynecologic cancer scare and knew that she needed to find a new way of relating to herself, her friends and family, and her work, especially since she wanted to make significant life changes.

Easier said than done. She was battling some problematic habits. Over the years, she had confused escapism with self-care, and this had manifested in heavy drinking. Given her family history of alcoholism, she was on a slippery slope with addiction, especially with a Pisces moon, which indicated her propensity to try to bypass pain.

With coaching, she learned the importance of slowing down and caring for her emotional health. This meant her tolerating difficult emotions without numbing out. By doing so, she deconstructed the identity she had built in the corporate world of being super tough and always able to push through, and this allowed her to embrace cyclical attunement as a path of health.

In doing so, she was able to tune in to her feelings and properly tend to them. This was especially important for her. In addition to recovering from a cancer scare she was navigating the tail end of her menopausal transition, a period often wrought with emotional upheaval due to sharp hormonal shifts.

Her increasing self-awareness supported her in establishing boundaries in relationships that previously had felt draining. She made other important changes too. Instead of numbing out on alcohol or by eating ice cream, she started drinking green juices. Wanting to feel even more energized, she transitioned to a more nourishing and plant-based diet, which aligned with both her body's needs and her personal values.

With these new habits in place, as she moved out of the fast-paced corporate world and into running her own business, she no longer needed to escape for relief. Instead she found herself investing in self-care that helped her step more deeply into her healing journey. In doing so, she transformed how she expressed her Aries sun and Pisces moon combination.

Astrology serves your health by helping you understand yourself so you can tailor your life and choices accordingly. Your health is directly influenced by your lifestyle, and when, like Sara, you make lifestyle changes on behalf of your goals, you influence your health outcomes.

The Natal Chart and Health

As an astrologer and a coach, helping clients digest their cosmic curriculum is one of my absolute favorite things to do.

How do I do this? I start by breaking down their natal chart.

Your natal chart, which represents a snapshot of the sky, shows the position of the planets at the moment of your birth relative to where you were born. It illuminates your specific symbiotic relationship with the cosmos, your disposition and proclivities, and, ultimately, your strengths as well as the challenges that ripple through your life. Knowing this, you can make behavior choices that affect your mind, body, and spirit in positive ways.

To begin, we'll review a brief explanation of astrological terminology and components, then we'll discuss how these components all come together to inform your health via your cosmic curriculum. This chapter offers *a lot* of information. Please don't feel like you need to get all of it now. You can revisit it as needed. Take your time and go slow. Integrate it bit by bit. The study and practice of astrology is an in-depth journey — for some, myself included, a lifelong one.

The Basics of Western Astrology: The Tropical Zodiac

The tropical zodiac is a directional phenomenon.

—Gemini Brett, from Astrology Hub interview

Cosmic health uses Western astrology, which is based on the tropical zodiac. Western astrology originated at a time when Earth was assumed to be at the center of the universe. Though obviously Earth revolves around the sun, astrology uses a geocentric perspective because it caters to our experience here on Earth and how things appear from our vantage point. If this feels strange, consider this: we say the sun rises and sets. But actually, Earth rotates on its axis from west to east, and this creates the *apparent* rising and setting of the sun. It's an optical illusion.

While the zodiac signs and the constellations are sometimes interchangeable, in the tropical zodiac they are *always* distinct from one another. The signs are named after the constellations, but, except for the sun, the stars themselves don't have a starring role in how the tropical zodiac works.

Here's why: the tropical zodiac is not based on the constellations but rather on the cycles created by Earth's two planes of motion: its daily rotation on its axis, and its annual revolution around the sun.

Tropical astrology is predicated on how the planes of these two motions—Earth's equator projected into space, known as "the celestial equator," and the path Earth takes around the sun, known as "the eclip-tic"—create a cyclical dance with the sun. If this sounds complicated, just think of it this way: these are the exact same cycles that create night, day, and the seasons—cycles our bodies are biologically wired to synchronize with.

As the following picture displays, the solstice points and equinox points extend in the cardinal directions—north, south, east, and west—from the center of the sun, the most important star.

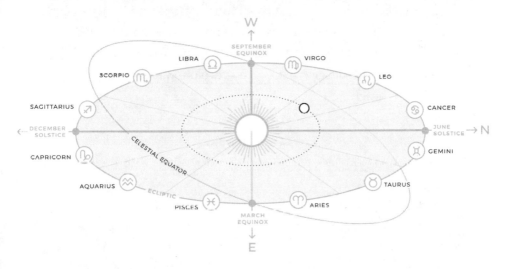

The seasons correspond with the cardinal directions, and they happen when:

1. The sun is due east of the center of Earth at zero degrees of Aries (March equinox)
2. The sun is due north of the center of Earth at zero degrees of Cancer (June solstice)

3. The sun is due west of the center of Earth at zero degrees of Libra (September equinox)
4. The sun is due south of the center of Earth at zero degrees of Capricorn (December solstice)[5]

Behind the ecliptic in a great circle—which is really an ellipse—are the constellations. But since the tropical zodiac and the constellations don't align, in tropical astrology, the ecliptic is divided into twelve equal thirty-degree segments, or the signs, starting with Aries and ending with Pisces. From a geocentric perspective, the sun appears to "move" along the ecliptic.

Astrologers refer to the sun as moving, but as I previously stated, it's not. A natal chart is *always* calculated from Earth; Earth is in the center of the chart. However, in the next set of images the sun is positioned in the center, with Earth moving around the sun. You can see based on the first two "flat" images that Earth's revolution around the sun puts the sun "in" a sign.

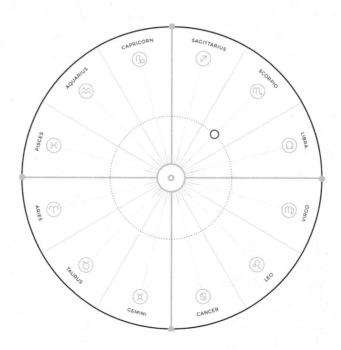

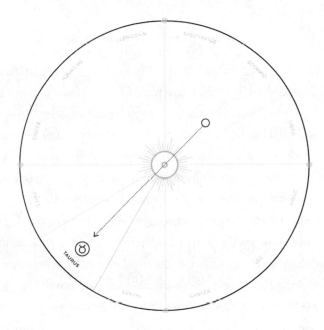

In this flat image you see Earth moving through the signs as they relate to the zodiacal year, which we will tackle next!

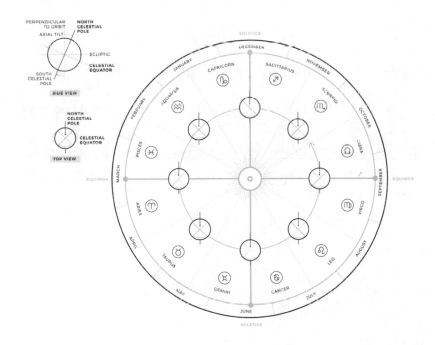

The Annual Zodiacal Year

As the starting point of the zodiacal year, zero degrees of Aries—the March equinox—is a time of renewal. The sun travels through Aries, then Taurus and Gemini. In the Northern Hemisphere, the June solstice, or the longest day of the year, occurs when the sun enters into Cancer; in the Southern Hemisphere, this is the shortest day of the year. Next up are Leo and Virgo. When we transition from Virgo into Libra, we cross the September equinox, and again we experience equal parts day and night, darkness and light. After the sign of Libra comes Scorpio, followed by Sagittarius. When the sun is due south of the center of the earth, we experience the December solstice, when the sun aligns with the Tropic of Capricorn and we enter Capricorn season. In the Northern Hemisphere, this brings the shortest day of the year, and in the Southern Hemisphere, the longest. From there, the sun's apparent movement traverses the signs of Capricorn, Aquarius, and Pisces, making its way back to Aries, where the zodiac begins again.

The Elements of the Zodiac

Each sign has both an element and a mode, which together determine how that sign expresses itself.

The elements speak to the four ways we categorize the astrological signs: earth, air, fire, and water. Since there are twelve signs, there are three signs per element, which is called "triplicity."

Fire (Aries, Leo, Sagittarius): Fire represents passion and vigor.

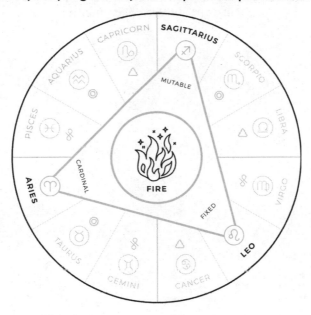

Earth (Taurus, Virgo, Capricorn): Earth represents grounded tenacity.

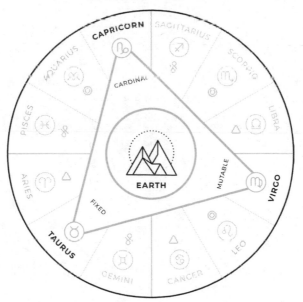

Air (Gemini, Libra, Aquarius): Air represents mental agility and analytical capacities.

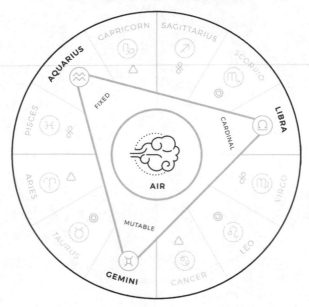

Water (Cancer, Scorpio, Pisces): Water represents emotional, intuitive, and empathetic capabilities.

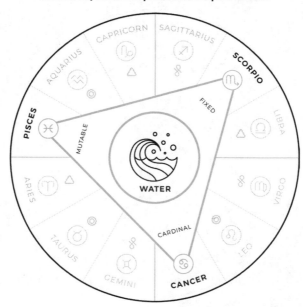

The Modes of the Zodiac

Each sign also has a mode, further defining its qualities: cardinal, fixed, or mutable. By following the movement of the sun and the succession of the seasons—spring, summer, fall, and winter—we find that each season encompasses a trio of signs, all following the same mode sequence, beginning with cardinal and moving into fixed and then mutable, in that order. The modes are referred to as the "quadruplicities," meaning four signs belong to each of the three distinct modes.

Cardinal (Aries, Cancer, Libra, Capricorn): Cardinal signs initiate a season. When the sun moves into these signs, we experience either a solstice or an equinox. Each of these seasons ushers in a new phase of the year, giving each sign a forcefulness and strong ability to initiate beginnings.

Fixed (Taurus, Leo, Scorpio, Aquarius): Fixed signs follow cardinal ones, and they bring stability to a season. Fixed signs temper the passion of cardinal signs, bringing steadfast focus, tenacity, and endurance.

Mutable (Gemini, Virgo, Sagittarius, Pisces): Mutable signs follow fixed signs and serve to facilitate transitions. They occur at the end of a season and provide a bridge from the fixed energy to the cardinal energy. They are adaptable and ready us for change.

Matching each element and mode, you'll find that there are twelve unique combinations, each attributed to a zodiac sign. In other words, no two zodiac signs have both the same element and mode. You'll also see that the elements and modes rotate in succession, creating a beautiful harmony over the course of each year.

Looking at each sign's element and mode together, we can honor our inherent complexity as humans. As just one example, Aquarius is an air sign (mentally agile and adept at change) yet fixed (focused, stable, sometimes even stubborn).

THE TWELVE SIGNS, THE ELEMENTS, AND THE MODES

Sign	Element	Mode	Dominant trait
♈ Aries	🔥 Fire	Cardinal	Initiatory
♉ Taurus	⛰ Earth	Fixed	Stabilizing
♊ Gemini	🌬 Air	Mutable	Versatile
♋ Cancer	🌊 Water	Cardinal	Tenacious
♌ Leo	🔥 Fire	Fixed	Inspired
♍ Virgo	⛰ Earth	Mutable	Industrious
♎ Libra	🌬 Air	Cardinal	Harmonious
♏ Scorpio	🌊 Water	Fixed	Mysterious
♐ Sagittarius	🔥 Fire	Mutable	Expansive
♑ Capricorn	⛰ Earth	Cardinal	Responsible
♒ Aquarius	🌬 Air	Fixed	Unconventional
♓ Pisces	🌊 Water	Mutable	Emotional

The Zodiac and the Body

Each astrological sign is also classically associated with certain areas of the human body. As we move sequentially through the zodiac, we travel from head to toe, with each sign's body part logically aligned with that sign's strengths and sensitivities. For instance, warm-hearted and brave Leo rules the back (especially the upper back) and heart—a strong spine and a full heart.

The signs correspond with the body's anatomical parts. The planets, however, also play a critical role and relate to the body's physiological functions.[6] (Medical astrology, when done well, is very nuanced and extremely specific.)

The following image shows the primary and traditional associations between the human body and the signs. The subsequent chart offers a

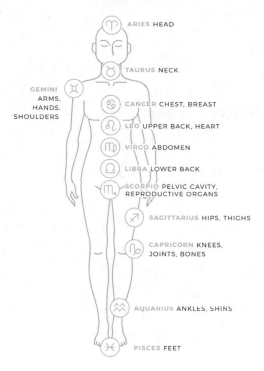

few more details, where necessary. This information is a jumping-off point to get started!

THE TWELVE SIGNS AND THE BODY

Sign	Element	Mode	Body part(s)
♈ Aries	🔥 Fire	Cardinal	Head, adrenals
♉ Taurus	⛰ Earth	Fixed	Throat, neck
♊ Gemini	☁ Air	Mutable	Hands, shoulders, arms, lungs
♋ Cancer	🌊 Water	Cardinal	Breast, stomach
♌ Leo	🔥 Fire	Fixed	Back, heart
♍ Virgo	⛰ Earth	Mutable	Small intestines, enteric nervous system, diaphragm
♎ Libra	☁ Air	Cardinal	Kidneys, lower back
♏ Scorpio	🌊 Water	Fixed	Sexual and reproductive organs, pelvic region

♐ Sagittarius	🔥 Fire	Mutable	Thighs, hips
♑ Capricorn	⛰ Earth	Cardinal	Knees, bones, skin, teeth
♒ Aquarius	💨 Air	Fixed	Ankles, shins, calves
♓ Pisces	🌊 Water	Mutable	Feet

The Planets and Luminaries

Because astrology subscribes to the wisdom of universal interconnectivity, we pay particular attention to all of the planets and the celestial bodies. However, the luminaries, the sun and the moon (which are also referred to as "planets" in astrology), have a stronger influence on our day-to-day experiences. The planets—Mercury, Venus, Mars, Jupiter, Saturn, Uranus, Neptune, and Pluto (in astrology we call Pluto a planet)—also play a significant role, which we will explore in part IV.

The planets follow their own cycles through the twelve astrological signs, with the length of their cycles dependent on each planet's speed and distance from the sun.

Each planet also has its own attributes and energy. How these attributes are expressed depends on which sign each planet is in within your natal chart (which we'll explore in depth in later chapters).

Each planet is also especially compatible with one or two signs. When the planets find themselves in the signs they "rule," they are at "home."

Similar to "The Twelve Signs and the Body," this list is by no means exhaustive. Here are the basics for your cosmic health journey.

THE PLANETS		
Planet	*Rules...*	*Attributes and energy*
☿ Mercury	Gemini, Virgo	Mindset, communication, intellect
♀ Venus	Taurus, Libra	Pleasure, love, values
♂ Mars	Aries, Scorpio	Desire, action, motivation

♃	Jupiter	Sagittarius, Pisces	Meaning, wisdom, abundance
♄	Saturn	Capricorn, Aquarius	Structure, discipline, productivity, time
♅	Uranus	Aquarius	Liberation, authenticity, creativity
♆	Neptune	Pisces	Spirituality, unity, illusion
♇	Pluto	Scorpio	Shadow, transmutation, birth, death

THE LUMINARIES		
Luminary	*Rules...*	*Attributes and energy*
☉ Sun	Leo	Identity, basic character, vitality
☾ Moon	Cancer	Emotions, desires, nurturance

Other Celestial Bodies

In addition to the planets and luminaries, other celestial bodies, including Chiron, Ceres, Juno, Vesta, and Pallas, may appear on your chart. As you become more familiar with the workings of your natal chart, you may want to look at the positions and signs of other celestial bodies as well.

This book focuses primarily on the eight planets, the two luminaries, and Chiron. Chiron is a comet-asteroid hybrid, known as a centaur. I included him in this book because he represents core wounds or wounds that never totally heal. After all, healing isn't always about resolving pain. Sometimes it's about developing the capacity to be with pain and developing compassion to help others, which is what Chiron teaches us to do.

The Twelve Houses

As you will see when you run your chart, your personal astrology is presented as a circle, or "pie," so to speak. That pie is divided into twelve slices, or houses.

What follows is a general description of each house. Like the signs and planets, this list is by no means exhaustive. Consider it a jumping-off point.

There are numerous house systems; the one I work with and will refer to throughout this book is Placidus, one of the most popular house systems.

First House: The first house cusp represents your rising sign. (A house cusp is the division point between two houses.) This house represents your body, how you express yourself, and your physical presentation to the world. The first house is particularly important when it comes to health since it represents your physical nature.

Second House: This house represents your sense of self-worth and your values, as well as most of your material possessions. It also indicates your financial affairs and habits. The second house relates to your health journey by demonstrating how you value yourself. Cultivating a deep sense of self-worth is critical to your healing journey. This is the work of the second house.

Third House: This house governs communication and writing. The third house relates to your local community, your early childhood development, and your siblings too. Therapy, journaling, and the ability to name and address issues are essential parts of your healing journey; understanding your third house helps you to activate the communication central to all of these.

Fourth House: This house represents your home or real estate, parents, and family roots. It's symbolic of what you need to feel safe and secure in your life, as well as your heritage. On the darker side of things, it correlates with endings. The fourth house cusp represents the imum coeli, or IC, of your chart. From the perspective of health, your fourth house shows how you relate to your foundation in life.

Fifth House: This house represents creativity, artistic expression, and children. The fifth house is associated with fun, pleasure, free time, dating, and romance. Since the fifth house represents recreation and the energy of fertility, this portion of your chart contributes to your health by supporting your vitality and creative self-expression.

Sixth House: This house, the house of service, represents your diet, health habits, daily actions, and day-to-day work. It's synonymous with routine, including seeing your medical professionals as needed and engaging in a movement practice that's appropriate for your constitution. The sixth house is one of the most critical houses when it comes to health. Your behaviors, lifestyle choices, and mindset contribute greatly to how your health manifests.

Seventh House: The cusp of the sixth and seventh houses is known as the descendant. This house represents both business and romantic relationships that are secured through contract (e.g., marriage). The seventh house also illuminates your "open enemies," such as competitors. Since relationships are a key indicator of longevity and health, this portion of your chart holds weight when it comes to partnering in ways that promote your best self.

Eighth House: This house represents shared resources—a partner's income, money earned through commissions, and anything having to do with credit, loans, inheritance, mortgages, etc. From a health perspective, this house represents the act of sex, primal desires, secrets, and the death-rebirth cycle. Wellness and the erotic are inevitably linked. Intimacy, both physical and emotional, is a critical foundation of health.

Ninth House: This house rules religion, higher education, big-picture thinking, publishing, and long-distance travel. Legal matters also belong to the ninth house. Faith remains a critical part of well-being, as does education. Keeping your brain inspired and motivated helps ward off cognitive stagnation and atrophy. The ninth house remains an important house on the path of self-actualization.

Tenth House: This house rules career, ambition, and honors. Beyond career status, the tenth house can also represent authorities, like your parents or your boss. The tenth house cusp, known as the midheaven or medium coeli (MC), is one of the most critical points of your chart. It signifies what you are known for via your social status and reputation, but it also indicates your aspirations and what lights you up from the perspective of a career path.

Eleventh House: This house represents your desires and ability to manifest them. Traditionally known as the house of friendship, it also rules groups, organizations, and acquaintances. Describing your personal and sometimes even professional goals, this house is essential to making your dreams a reality. It's about your aspirations, affiliations, and social connections—an important part of life that motivates your desire for well-being and high-performance living.

Twelfth House: This house rules your subconscious and aspects of life that are hidden. Closely associated with the occult, it traditionally represents self-undoing. While it can be associated with addiction, from an evolved perspective this house offers an invitation to spiritual wisdom and metaphysical tenacity. The twelfth house is a mysterious house. Its essence is about spiritual reflection, privacy, and what's beneath the surface, all of which contribute to health.

Throughout this book, I help you get to know the planets through the signs, but I don't offer interpretations for house placements. In the resource section in the appendix you will find book recommendations for further study.

The Astrological Aspects

Aspects refer to the angular relationship, or positioning, of the planets at any given moment in time, showing how their respective energies are connecting and relating to one another.

Here's a basic overview of the aspects:

☌ **Conjunction (0°):** when two planets merge with each other, blending their strengths, and initiating a new cycle

⚹ **Sextile (60°):** a harmonious and supportive blend of power supporting the growth of new endeavors

☐ **Square (90°):** a cosmic clash expediting growth and commanding focus

△ **Trine (120°):** a manifestation of support, indicating a gift or harmonious interactions

⚻ **Quincunx (150°):** leaning into discomfort as a path to purpose; incongruities that suggest a need for reconciliation

☍ **Opposition (180°):** peak tensions bringing issues to the surface; a culmination of power

Bringing It All Together

The Natal Chart vs. Transits

It's essential to know the difference between a natal chart (the chart based on the date, place, and time of birth), which is a static chart—it doesn't change—and planetary transits. Transits reflect where the planets are today and their continuous shifting. Transits act like a weather report for what is happening now and what will happen in the future. In part II we'll discuss the transits of the moon and the sun, while in parts III and IV we'll look at how the planets animate themselves in your natal chart.

Don't have a chart? At JenniferRacioppi.com/resources I have supplemental free ebook to support the integration of what you will learn in this book, including a brief overview of my favorite places online to access your chart for free, as well as additional information about the signs, the planets, and your body.

Astrology, Health, and Personal Transformation

Mari is one of many great examples of how astrology influences health.

A single, Black, college-educated woman living in New York City who'd worked in hospitality for years as a bartender, Mari yearned to live a more expressed version of herself. She wanted a new and different life, one that felt aligned with who she was at the deepest level. The problem was, the life she desired, the one she could see, feel, and taste in her mind, seemed so far removed from the life she was living, she wasn't sure her dreams of better health, a loving relationship, and a more fulfilling career were actually possible. However, she also knew she'd never forgive herself if she didn't go for her boldest hopes and dreams.

Mari was, without a doubt, one of the hardest-working clients I've ever had. The commitment, determination, and energy she brought to the process was no accident. Having lost her mom years prior to cancer, she understood the impermanence of life and felt a sense of urgency to live the life she wanted. She was so ready to transform her life that she was able to tap into divine timing, which gave her additional momentum to create the many changes she desired.

However, making the needed changes felt hard, especially at first. For years Mari had lived a party lifestyle and was hanging out with people who reinforced the behaviors that kept her stuck. That made a lot of sense, given her chart. With a Gemini sun (super social, always on the go), a natal moon in Leo (deep need to be seen, to be in the mix), and Sagittarius rising (seeks total freedom, rejects rules), she was prone to pursuing the next thrill, which temporarily elevated her energy. But going to another gathering filled with people who always wanted to party was leading her away from, rather than toward, the life she truly desired. She wanted professional success. She wanted a spiritual discipline and a life partner. She wanted to feel strong and fit, not hungover and constantly behind on her goals.

On top of these mental anguishes, physically she suffered from endometriosis. Her late nights at work, where she ate bar food and ended her shift with a drink, kept her in a cycle that zapped her confidence and made her pain even worse. Determined to feel better, Mari began a lifestyle overhaul.

As a Gemini sun sign, Mari used the mind–body practice of yoga to help calm her overactive, ruminative thinking, reducing her anxiety. But it was a struggle. Being such a naturally social pleasure-seeker, she struggled with putting her phone away for a full hour. To her, that felt like sensory and social deprivation—a heart-wrenchingly lonely experience. She felt similarly isolated when she began to pull away from the people keeping her stuck in her old, party-centric lifestyle. In spite of these challenges, Mari persevered, not just with yoga and working out, both of which helped her enormously, but also with significant adjustments to her diet.

In addition to coaching with me, she read countless books on personal development. She was, as I like to say, drinking from the spiritual fire-hose, night and day, soaking up any and all wisdom and guidance she could find.

Because she was able to make these changes, she began to experience the benefits of a rested, nourished body. While this alone did not eradicate her endometriosis, it certainly reduced unnecessary stress on her body and supported her endocrine system immensely. With these new habits in place, not only did she transition her job but she also found within herself the capacity to cultivate intimate trust in her closest relationship, which led to a radical reinvention of self. All of this combined meant she had less pain and more peace, and lost fewer days to feeling hungover.

Eight years later, Mari is married to a partner with whom she shares a deep connection. She transitioned out of working in hospitality. Her first job after bartending was event planning, and since then she has become a senior director at a creative agency working in advertising. She now lives in a penthouse and enjoys a healthier relationship with her body. She's integrated cosmic health into her life in ways that continue to support her.

Syncing with the Sun and the Moon

While we'll eventually discuss how to sensitize ourselves to the cycles of distant planets like Uranus and Pluto, the lunisolar cycles have the greatest impact on the biological rhythms that influence our health, our development, and, thus, our lives.

Now that we've looked at the basic elements of astrology and health, as well as the natal chart, we'll focus on these core aspects—beginning with the lunar cycle and how it affects health and well-being.

Part II

EARTH

Embracing the Magic of Cyclical Living

As the moon formed about 4.51 billion years ago, life evolved equally under both lunar and solar influences and might have adapted multiple times to moon rhythms to coordinate complex processes.
—Gabriele Andreatta and Kristin Tessmar-Raible, from "The Still Dark Side of the Moon: Molecular Mechanisms of Lunar-Controlled Rhythms and Clocks"

CHAPTER 3

Living in Sync with
Lunar Cycles

Healer Debbie Lefay, my first spiritual mentor, taught me the art of lunar ritual. But it was Freedom Cole, my yoga teacher and Vedic astrologer, who taught me how to live in sync with the moon for daily health. I started working with Freedom at a time when everything in my life felt chaotic. I had just moved to San Francisco, alone, to finish college. And then, a few weeks later, 9/11 happened. Struggling to establish a routine on a shoestring budget in a new city where I didn't know anyone, amidst a global crisis, and while still adjusting to my postmenopausal body was downright anxiety-provoking.

"If you get a calendar that outlines the moon's daily transits, you'll start to understand the moon's impact on your emotions," he told me at the start of our work together. That, he explained, would allow me to predict monthly fluctuations in my mood and symptoms, helping me to better manage my anxiety. As I anticipated those fluctuations, I'd be able to take care of myself preemptively. It was eye-opening, and it gave me hope.

I immediately began tracking my emotions and physical symptoms in a journal, including descriptions of daily lunar transits and other astrological events. When I combined this with the knowledge I had learned from Debbie, I soon realized that I always felt my best at the new moon and my worst at the full moon. By marrying this knowledge with my self-care practices, I began to connect to a new monthly rhythm.

Knowing that each new moon offered a new beginning, I always had something to look forward to. Each month I celebrated the new moon with the same earnestness that most people only conjure for New Year's Eve. I also constructed an altar in a small corner of my apartment where I could meditate and perform my rituals. This practice became nonconventional mind–body medicine that helped to calm my nervous system as I integrated my healing.

I got clear on what I needed each month to advance my healing. In addition to my new moon ritual, I followed up with a minimum of three rituals to navigate the rest of the lunar cycle — one each for the waxing phase, the full moon phase, and the waning phase. Each week, I focused on a different aspect of the lunar cycle, and with every ritual, I felt more connected to what I needed to heal.

With this new understanding of how I experienced the lunar-regulated rhythm of my emotions and my body, I stopped expecting to feel good all the time. My emotions were cyclical and, therefore, impermanent. I could feel intensely melancholy or frustrated or afraid yet also trust that those feelings would pass. Further, by syncing my life to the moon's phases, I could conjure my will and work with the moon's rhythm to create radical lifestyle shifts—this was game-changing.

As I became healthier emotionally, I felt more optimistic and hopeful, which motivated me to take better care of myself physically. That meant practicing yoga, eating unprocessed foods, and going to therapy. I also quickly figured out that doing all the right things didn't lead to feeling all of the right feelings all of the time. I could break down, have bad days — and still grow stronger and more resilient.

These are just some of the gifts that the moon has given me, and my clients too.

In this chapter, we'll look at the different phases of the lunar cycle and see how to tap into them to bolster our emotional well-being and get what we want in our health and our lives.

The Root of Health and Happiness

Ruled astrologically by the moon and the sign of Cancer, our emotions are the foundation of our health. These are two guiding principles of my work as a coach and an astrologer:

- Our emotional awareness is a fundamental, but often overlooked, basis of our healing.
- Our emotional health doesn't just help us heal physically; it is the fertile ground in which every relationship, every dream, and everything we desire can and must grow.

Why? Because when we *feel* better, we *do* better.

When we value ourselves, we're more willing to tend to our physical health—by prioritizing sleep, a nutritious diet, exercise, self-care, and more.

When we feel better, we're more willing to take action toward realizing our bigger dreams.

When we feel better, we thrive in our relationships—with ourselves, our loved ones, our friends, our family, and even with money.

When we tend to our emotional center, we gain access to an abundance of passion, which we can then utilize on behalf of the reclamation of our power. This helps us to heal ourselves, our lives, and the world around us.

But first, we must tend to our inner world. This isn't just my experience and opinion; it's also science. Nearly a century ago, Freud discovered that repressed emotion leads to physical symptoms. More recent studies have found that over 80 percent of doctor visits involve a social/emotional issue, with only 16 percent regarding matters purely physical in nature.[1]

The lesson here? Before all else, we must heal how we feel.

What Is Emotional Health?

Emotional health refers to how we manage our thoughts and feelings. Each of us cycles through tens of thousands of unique thoughts each day, and many of them are rooted in emotion. How we process, express, and behave in the context of our thoughts and feelings contributes to our emotional health.

Let's pause briefly to digest this—because emotional health isn't just about having positive thoughts, feeling good, and being happy. Contrary to popular psychology, which commands us to "be happy" and "think positive," the science of positive psychology encourages us to feel and process our darker, more challenging emotions fully and honestly, not to mask, suppress, or inhibit how we feel. While being with what hurts, we develop a capacity to accept and learn from pain. In doing so, we learn adaptive ways to handle the inevitable hardships of life, and we grow more resilient.[2]

Tending to our emotional health therefore means embracing the inevitable ebbs and flows of our lives. We can't rush through unpleasant emotions, like fear, grief, or sadness. To be emotionally healthy, we can't use forced positive thinking to avoid feeling angry or heartbroken. Instead, we have to give our emotions—*all* of them—the time and space they need to be expressed and then to evolve.

Feeling the full range and force of our emotions is central to our physical health as well. In fact, emotional health and physical health are interwoven—remember, *everything is connected.* A person can be in good enough physical shape to run a marathon yet so stressed out that her sleep and digestion are suffering. That's because how we handle our emotions affects our physical well-being. We also see this phenomenon occur in reverse: strong emotional health correlating with desired physical health outcomes.

Beyond our physical constitution, emotional wellness guides behavior and decision-making that can have lasting consequences on our physical, social, and professional worlds.

So how do we handle our emotions, especially since they often seem mysterious, out of our control, even unwanted?

Accessing Your Emotions

To relate to our emotions in more empowering ways, we first need to be clear about how we're feeling. As we rush through our busy days, perpetually distracted by technology, that's sometimes easier said than done. If nothing else, tuning out our emotions can be a habit that takes effort to break.

Here's a simple exercise you can try to connect with yourself. Quickly scan your mind, body, and emotions, and evaluate what's happening for you, in this moment. Ask yourself: What am I feeling? What am I thinking? What do I need? Give yourself time for your feelings, thoughts, and intuitive wisdom to arrive. If you feel numb or unaware, know this: just because your emotions aren't readily available doesn't mean they aren't there. Often, the body stops feeling as a way to self-protect. So be patient and give yourself the time that your feelings need to surface. Then, acknowledge what they are communicating. If it's appropriate, take action on the directives you are receiving from your body, mind, and spirit.

The Beauty of Impermanence

In those moments when our emotions feel bigger and more powerful than we are, we forget one critical fact: when we let ourselves feel emotions fully, their intensity peaks, and while they may feel like they will last forever, they won't. By feeling our emotions, we give ourselves the opportunity to let them go and feel other ones.

In ancient Buddhist practices, this process of continuous evolution is referred to as "impermanence." Everything and everyone experiences birth and death; nothing is meant to stay the same or last forever. A moment is only ever supposed to be a moment—no more.

The same goes for our emotions. By allowing ourselves to experience the good and the bad, the easy and the hard, we heal.

No cosmic influence exemplifies impermanence and novelty more beautifully than the moon herself. The moon is constantly changing from new to full, waning, and so on. She also moves through a different zodiac sign approximately every two and a half days. Yet always, like you, she remains herself, even as she changes. The moon's cyclical nature exemplifies how to move from darkness to light while journeying through different experiences each time.

The Moon: Some Scientific Facts

Moon phases are created by the moon's revolution around Earth, relative to the sun. Remember, the moon doesn't have light unto itself. As it revolves around Earth it cyclically changes its position to the sun, reflecting an evolving intensity of the sun's light back to us.

The moon's gravitational pull controls the ocean tides. However, the ocean has its strongest tides, spring tides, when the moon is either new or full, when the sun's gravitational impact magnifies this effect. Since our bodies are composed of 50–75 percent water, many believe this same gravitational phenomenon also affects us as humans.

Though the gravitational impact controlling the tides is scientifically debated as having an influence on human behavior, there's evidence emerging in the field of chronobiology to suggest that humans might also have endogenous biological rhythms similar to the circadian rhythm that work "circa-monthly." Endogenous biological rhythms function independent of external cues but work best when synchronized with the external light–dark cycle they adaptively mirror. The circadian rhythm is endogenous. Another hypothesis is that humans don't have a cira-monthly clock but are simply driven by external cues, such as the shifting light at night associated with moon-phase changes.[3]

Whether or not humans have innate biological clocks that work in rhythm with the moon, it's a well-known scientific fact that many animals and plants do. I'm excited to see what emerges in the research on this topic in the years ahead. I have a hunch that there's a lot to learn!

The Moon: Your Guide and Confidante

Lunar energy, always engaging in its near-monthly cycle of waxing and waning, bestows a cycle that we can harness as a gateway to initiation and manifestation.

By understanding the nuances of the moon's transits through the zodiac, you'll learn how to feel your emotions in a healthy and productive way—and then use them to unearth your own healing momentum.

Syncing with the Moon's Phases to Enhance Your Emotional Health

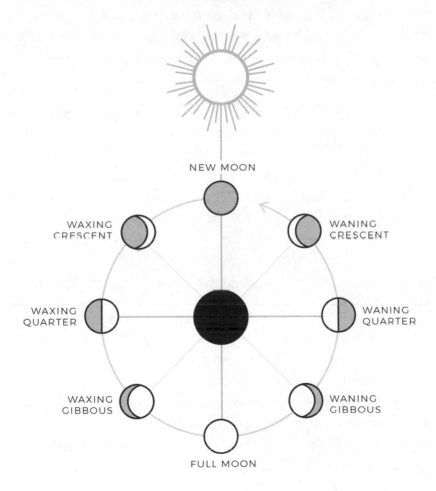

NEW MOON

WAXING CRESCENT

WANING CRESCENT

WAXING QUARTER

WANING QUARTER

WAXING GIBBOUS

WANING GIBBOUS

FULL MOON

Following the moon's cycle is the absolute best way to begin to learn astrology, understand your body's cyclical shifts and your emotional needs, and improve your well-being. There are eight lunar phases to consider.

New Moon: The new moon occurs when the sun and moon align at the same degree. We generally have one new moon per month, though occasionally we have no new moon or two new moons in one month. Because it takes twenty-nine-and-a-half days to transit between new moons, they occur on different days each month.

Each new moon brings a dark night with no visible moon in the sky. Emotionally, a new moon is the time to tune in to your heart's desires. This is a powerful opportunity to set new intentions and actively choose to meet your deeper longings. Now's the time to ascertain your needs and make a commitment to calling in your desires.

Waxing Crescent: Immediately after a new moon, as the moon starts to move out of direct alignment with the sun, it begins to wax, giving us a glimpse of a slender crescent in the night sky. This is commonly referred to as Diana's bow. This is the time to take action on the seeds of intention that you planted at the new moon. Notice how you feel during the transition from the new moon to the waxing crescent moon. For example, do you feel focused and energized? Drained and anxious? Ambivalent and unaware? Start to track this. This part of the moon's cycle encourages follow-through on intentions set with the new moon.

Waxing Quarter: The waxing quarter moon happens when the sun and moon square, making a ninety-degree angle to each other. This occurs at the halfway point between the new moon and full moon. A waxing quarter moon looks like a half moon and indicates a period of transition. Often bringing creative opportunities, it's the time to commit to your desires. However, the square between the sun and the moon also indicates a need for reconciliation of unseen obstacles, so dig deeper into your intentions and know that unanticipated curveballs may arise.

◐ *Waxing Gibbous:* After the waxing quarter moon, the moon begins to look fuller each night. With the sun and the moon in a harmonious relationship at this point in the lunar cycle, you may feel energized, on point, and goal driven. This phase of the moon asks you to commit to your grit. Remember Angela Duckworth's definition that I cited in chapter 1? Grit is a combination of passion and perseverance. This phase of the moon invites a steadfast approach to achieving your goals. However, the brighter and fuller light and lunar energy at this time can also lead to insomnia and restlessness.[4] Observing how you respond around this time can help you understand and anticipate the cyclical patterns of your individual well-being.

◯ *Full Moon:* When the sun and moon oppose each other in the sky, the moon reflects the sun's light back to Earth, making it appear full. Astrologically, during this moon phase, the sun and the moon always occupy opposite zodiac signs, which may bring a sense of heightened creativity and, sometimes, feelings of tension. Full moons offer the opportunity to see what is not working in your life so you can begin to make changes. They also expedite the manifestation of goals. Because of the extra light at night, your daily rhythms may be affected, shifting your sleep cycles and your energy. By paying extra attention to how you feel during the full moon, you can adjust your self-care accordingly.

◑ *Waning Gibbous:* Immediately after the full moon, the moon begins to wane. This is a time, ideally, to finish things. Check in and evaluate where you can pull back and surrender. Listen to the voice of your soul, and allow it to guide you. Also notice what is coming to fruition in your life. What has manifested? What are you still desiring and what is standing in your way? Pay close attention to your physical state. How do you feel in your body? What is shifting in your emotional state? How social do you feel?

◑ *Waning Quarter:* At this time the moon looks like a half moon but is actually a quarter moon. Similar to the waxing quarter moon, a waning quarter moon appears when the sun and moon square, or form a disharmonious ninety-degree angle with each other. This is a moment to weed the proverbial garden. Resolve issues and complete projects. Lean into any discomfort you feel. As the moon's light wanes, this phase synergistically invites you to release what is no longer serving you. Consequently, this portion of the moon's cycle often reveals intentions from long ago presently coming to fruition too.

Waning Crescent: This introspective moment of the lunar cycle is a good time to review what you've learned since the new moon. What intention did you set? What progress have you made since? Looking back on the previous weeks to assess what you learned helps you consider your intentions for the upcoming lunar cycle. The moon is waning dark now, which may make you feel a bit lethargic, tired, or withdrawn. It's also common to feel a bit melancholy. Use this time to grieve and rest! A "dark moon" can be defined as the three-day period before a new moon. Often experienced as the most challenging time of the cycle, it teaches you how to gracefully surrender, accept your emotional truth, and hear the voice of your intuition. This is a time to connect to the void, the metaphorical experience of "chaos."

A Brief (but Necessary) Dose of Reality

When I started tracking the moon's phases as a daily practice, I was a twentysomething college student—which is to say poor in funds but rich in time.

Keep in mind, there are many unique and empowering ways to integrate the lunar cycle into your life that don't require a lot of time. Heather, who's been a coaching client of mine for years, is a great example of this.

Heather, a mid-thirties white female entrepreneur living in the Midwest, is forever juggling her clientele, multiple employees, and an incredibly packed schedule. With her natal sun in Capricorn, it's no surprise that Heather relies on routines and discipline to stay healthy and productive. From her exercise schedule to her food and more, each week is a fine-tuned machine that works best *without* variation and *with* absolute consistency and precision. Her regimented lifestyle is what allows her to do everything she needs to do each week.

Even during the early days of the COVID-19 crisis, when her gym closed, she did circuit training in her house every morning for thirty minutes. Not only did this help her stay emotionally steady during the chaotic times she faced in business, but also her daily movement practice helps her keep her knees healthy. (She has minor knee problems, a common Capricorn issue.) Movement allows her to stay pain-free.

Not wanting to compromise her sacred regimen, Heather uses the lunar cycle in very specific ways. By staying aware of how the lunar phases affect her energy, she now knows when to add bits of unscheduled time to her calendar (these quieter times are great for creativity and big-picture thinking). When she's likely to feel social, she focuses more of her time and energy on networking and attending events. She also integrates her personal astrology into how she shows up as a leader and in her intimate relationship.

While these changes may seem small in the context of her incredibly hectic schedule, they have added up to a huge shift in her outlook and energy. While her free time is still sparse, by honoring her emotional ebbs and flows and the lunar phases, Heather has been able to tend to more of her needs and desires in her business and personal life. She's also come to appreciate the times each month, usually during the dark moon, when she can carve out periods of quiet, allowing her to be with and feel the excruciating grief she's experienced since losing her sister to cancer.

By honoring the natural rhythms of the lunar phases, we leverage our peak productivity periods and engage in deep rest and recovery when it's called for. When we know how to tap into this natural cycle, creating the life we want becomes a lot easier.

The Moon through the Zodiac

Now that we've looked at some of the many ways we can integrate lunar rhythms as a cornerstone in our cyclical living practices to boost our health and well-being, let's look at the moon's transits through each of the zodiac signs.

As mentioned previously, the moon traverses in and out of each zodiac sign approximately every two-and-a-half days. This is slightly longer than two lunar days—it takes the moon 24.8 hours to revolve around Earth. By tracking the moon through the signs, we learn to acknowledge, understand, and express our feelings with cyclical attunement to the zodiac. You may find that you feel differently depending on which sign the moon is in at any given time. Track your experience based on where the moon is in the zodiac, and you'll develop a deeper understanding of your emotional well-being and when to focus on different types of self-care.

TRACKING THE MOON

You can track the moon through its phases using various resources:

Since 1818, **Farmers' Almanac** has been a trusted knowledge base for long-term weather and astronomical tracking, for timing activities in the home and the earth. The official website offers both a moon-phase and a moon-sign calendar (farmersalmanac .com/calendar/moon-phases/; farmersalmanac.com/calendar /zodiac/).

The **Café Astrology** home page is typically updated with the day's moon details and notable transits. You can also check out their moon phase calendar (cafeastrology.com/calendars/moon phasescalendar.html) and get a snapshot of the present transits with an online calculator (cafeastrology.com/current-astrological -transits.html).

MoonSign.Today has a moon calendar available online as well as free and paid versions of moon-tracking software for your computer (moonsign.today).

An **ephemeris** is a table, data file, or reference book used to track the movement of celestial bodies and is a critical astrological tool that will show you the daily position of each planet as well as the moon. (The plural of *ephemeris* is *ephemerides*.)

Astrology software like Solar Fire offers calendars with details of the moon's (and other planets') transits.

An increasing number of moon-tracking **phone apps** have hit the market. If this is more your style for checking in on the moon, I encourage you to look for an app you like (and remember to check its reputability!).

Note: The following are general descriptions of the moon's transit through each sign, so they're *not* specific to any natal chart. In addition to a general description of each moon, I've included a summary of each new and full moon, and again, these are not specific to any natal chart. At the time of the new moon, the sun and moon are always in the same sign. At the time of a full moon, the sun and moon are always in signs opposite each other. Each month we all experience what's known as a lunar return, which is when the moon returns to our natal moon sign. At this time, there's an alignment between our natal lunar predisposition and what's happening astrologically in the sky.

Moon in Aries ♈

As a cardinal fire sign and the first sign of the zodiac, Aries ushers in fiery energy, action, growth, and new beginnings. When the moon is in Aries, step into leadership on behalf of your dreams. Tap into your emotional need for action and independence to ramp up the momentum in your life.

New Moon in Aries: The new moon in Aries is the first new moon of the astrological year, the March equinox, making it *extra* important. Aries initiates new beginnings with ferocity. It invites you to explore your passions. Since Mars rules Aries, it's a potent new moon for initiating a movement or exercise practice.

Full Moon in Aries: A full moon in Aries occurs at the Aries-Libra axis, inviting you to acknowledge the dichotomy of me versus us. It encourages introspection around relationships, especially issues stemming from codependency and people pleasing. This, too, is a potent time to exercise and practice the releasing of anger.

Moon in Taurus ♉

Taurus is a fixed earth sign that emphasizes your need for loyalty, embodiment, and steadfast commitment to your desired outcomes. Balancing practicality with beauty and sensuality, this feel-good sign can also resist change—which isn't always a bad thing. When the moon is in Taurus, dig your heels into the earth and get grounded. Eat for nourishment, move your body for pleasure, and stay committed to your goals.

New Moon in Taurus: This new moon evokes a connection to sensuality and sexuality. Slow down, feel the sensations in your body, and give voice to your needs. What you begin on this new moon sticks, so consider starting a meditation practice (if you don't already have one) or any other discipline that provides mind–body healing.

Full Moon in Taurus: A Taurus full moon highlights the Scorpio-Taurus axis, marking a precious opportunity to experience lunar-charged, full-blown embodiment and connection to sexuality. It encourages you to explore the dichotomy between security (Taurus) and risk (Scorpio). Focus on pleasure, play, and sensuality. Be open to speaking and receiving the truth.

Moon in Gemini ♊

Gemini is a mutable air sign that fuels your mental agility, ideas, and creativity. Communication in its many forms—writing, talking, journaling, and anything that facilitates the cross-pollination of ideas—is favored. When the moon is in Gemini, connect with people and ideas in unique ways, and in the process, enable collaborative leadership.

New Moon in Gemini: With a new moon in Gemini, you may find yourself bursting with new ideas and possibilities. While this new moon might feel a bit ungrounded, it's essential to write out your hopes, goals, dreams, and wishes, especially as they relate to self-expression or healing. This is a great new moon for initiating talk therapy or any other healing modality that involves self-expression.

Full Moon in Gemini: Partnered with the sun in Sagittarius, a full moon in Gemini represents a need for mental stimulation, freedom, exploration, and growth. Whether you seek social experiences or choose to engage your curiosity with intriguing books, keep your head, heart, and ears open for fresh and different perspectives. Look at where you feel held back in your life and choose actions that allow you to feel the essence of liberation.

Moon in Cancer ♋

Cancer, a cardinal water sign ruled by the moon, represents the sacred feminine, your ancestry, and your desire for safety, comfort, and security. Because Cancer is a loving, nurturing, and healing sign that rules emotions, when the moon is in Cancer, do things that help build your self-esteem.

New Moon in Cancer: This is a wonderful new moon in which to set intentions to heal family dynamics, current-day issues, or issues stemming from your bloodline's history. Beckoning you to explore your needs for safety and security, this time is also opportune for planting seeds of financial abundance. As you do, embrace the vulnerability that accompanies intimacy.

Full Moon in Cancer: Partnered with the sun in Capricorn, a Cancer full moon promotes working industriously toward the accomplishment of your life goals...in your slippers and robe. Under this full moon, you could receive insights on your relationship with family, especially your parents, or children if you are a parent. Use this full moon to appreciate what you love about your family and bring mindful attention to the patterns that no longer serve you so you can surrender.

Moon in Leo ♌

A fixed fire sign, Leo is playful, confident, generous, and creative. Leo energy helps you show up authentically while letting others shine as well. Under the moon in Leo, give yourself praise and attention. What's going well for you? Acknowledge your strengths with gratitude and reflect on how you can use them even more.

New Moon in Leo: During this new moon, set intentions to grow through play, live with courage, and embrace your leadership. See yourself for who you really are: a divine creature with a purpose. This new moon is an invitation to reinvigorate your vitality and self-determination.

Full Moon in Leo: This full moon activates the Aquarius-Leo axis, awakening your individuality and playfulness. Listen to the needs of your inner child. As you align with your truth, you may feel more courageous. If this seems scary, feel the fear and keep moving forward anyway.

Moon in Virgo ♍

A mutable earth sign, Virgo is oriented toward service, refinement, and precision as well as systemization and productivity. Under a moon in Virgo, awaken to the healthiest version of yourself and your environment.

Instead of striving for perfection, aim for consistent action. Embrace structure, get organized and clean, and focus on maintaining the healthy behaviors that allow you to feel strong. Carve out alone time, which is essential during a Virgo moon.

> **New Moon in Virgo:** This new moon asks you to look at your health and craft a vision of how you want to feel and which self-care practices support that. It initiates a return to personal sovereignty, greater alignment with your truth, and a vision for your healthiest, most radiant life. Look at dynamics in your life that have dimmed your power, and set an intention to take your power back.
>
> **Full Moon in Virgo:** A full moon in Virgo activates the Pisces-Virgo axis. This is the most monastic moon of them all—a time to simplify and streamline. This is a great chance to recommit to basic healthy eating habits, like eating a blood-sugar balancing diet, consuming lots of leafy greens, and drinking plenty of water. You may crave alone time. If so, give yourself the space you desire.

Moon in Libra ♎

As a cardinal air sign, the moon in Libra inspires action. During a Libra moon, ask yourself what in your life feels in or out of balance. Where are you mistreating yourself? Libra values fairness and harmony, so confronting conflict and owning darker emotions, while challenging, is also important now. Similarly, Libra highlights justice, asking you to align with your values and stand up for your truth.

> **New Moon in Libra:** This new moon invites you to set intentions for justice, harmony, and peace. Libra amplifies the healing power of self-expression through art while asking you to evaluate your relationships as well. Do the give and take in your relationships feel balanced? Get in touch with your personal values and consider how you can more fully commit to what truly matters.

Full Moon in Libra: This moon highlights the Aries-Libra axis and the push-pull between independence and your relationship with the greater good. This cardinal full moon may feel uncompromising. Commit to self-compassion. Use this full moon to tap into your creativity. Since the full moon is ruled by Venus, it's a time to reconnect with your values.

Moon in Scorpio ♏

Scorpio is a fixed water sign symbolizing ambition, independence, and a strong determination to excel. Dedicated to profound truth, Scorpio underscores the need for deep transformation. Find the meaning in darkness by exploring complicated ideas and emotions lurking in the shadows. Under a Scorpio moon, there is a high standard for authenticity. Scorpio also relates to sexuality, so check in and ask what you need in that area of your life.

New Moon in Scorpio: This new moon asks you to look at where you are holding back your truth and healing so you can welcome transformation. It asks you to get in touch with your sexuality; orgasm is critical for rejuvenation, vitality, stress relief, and even better sleep. Like the phoenix who rises from its ashes, a Scorpio new moon invites resurrection and transformation.

Full Moon in Scorpio: A full moon activates the Scorpio-Taurus axis. It represents a call to be in your body: tapped in and turned on. While this full moon may elicit emotional intensity, this is a great opportunity to channel it on behalf of what you intend to create in your life. Pay attention to secrets being revealed. While you may not agree with life's lessons, accepting them, with humility, expedites your healing process.

Moon in Sagittarius ♐

Sagittarius is a mutable fire sign that activates the urge for independence, big-picture ideas, adventure, travel, and philosophy. It embodies a love of learning, teaching, exploring, growing, and throwing out rules to honor truth. Because of this, a moon in Sagittarius may encourage you to say whatever is on your mind. Follow your instincts. You may also feel a need to exercise more during this time.

New Moon in Sagittarius: As one of the most visionary signs of the zodiac, Sagittarius turns thought into action. Although this new moon occurs during the holiday season, this is one of the best times to kick-start your workout routine. Asking you to restructure and reinvigorate how you relate to your vision for the future, this new moon provides an opportunity to seed new beginnings for hope, optimism, and growth.

Full Moon in Sagittarius: This full moon activates the Gemini-Sagittarius axis. Your freedom-seeking, adventurous spirit may be rallied by the potent energy of a full moon in Sagittarius. Experiment with what freedom means to you: push up against boundaries that hold you back, and seek out adventure. Speak your truth.

Moon in Capricorn ♑

Tenacious like no other, Capricorn, a cardinal earth sign, has a nose-to-the-grindstone work ethic that's all about getting things done. Capricorn energy encourages you to get serious and stay practical. This is a time to roll up your sleeves and get to work on behalf of your goals. Under this moon, notice how you can leverage structure and routine on behalf of your healing journey.

New Moon in Capricorn: A new moon in Capricorn, a sign known for perseverance, offers a robust opportunity to commit to your purpose. Things may feel serious and you may be driven to do it all—remember, you don't have to do it all alone. This new moon asks you to set ambitious goals and initiate new beginnings.

Full Moon in Capricorn: This full moon activates the Cancer-Capricorn axis, calling forth your inner boss. Beware of power struggles and execute your vision with practicality and compassion. Emotions and sensitivities may run high. Stand in your power, but check the power trip at the door. Ruled by Saturn, this full moon asks you to own your purpose, but also honor grief.

Moon in Aquarius ♒

An innovator and trendsetter, Aquarius isn't afraid to ditch convention and break the rules. Unlike Capricorn, Aquarius questions the effectiveness of tunnel-vision determination and focus around work. Instead, this fixed air sign underscores the need for change and the betterment of society. Under an Aquarius moon, stay open to heeding your intuition and honoring progressive visions. Creativity can lead you toward innovation. This is a heady time, so it's also important to be mindful of your emotions, which are here to guide you and keep you from becoming aloof.

> **New Moon in Aquarius:** This new moon is a time to unleash your uniqueness, authenticity, radical ideas, and creative leadership. Recommit to changes you wish to make, especially as they apply to your ideals, your community, and the thoughtful use of technology. Igniting a passion for social justice, a new moon in Aquarius provides an opportunity to set intentions for collective health. Develop and commit to a vision for your most desired future.
>
> **Full Moon in Aquarius:** An Aquarius full moon activates the Leo-Aquarius axis. You may feel inspired to notice where you needlessly conform to things that rob you of vitality, well-being, and individuality. It's time to embrace your eclecticism—even if that means clashing with the status quo. This is also a great time for fitness classes, group therapy, or attending support groups with like-minded people.

Moon in Pisces ♓

The final sign of the zodiac, Pisces is a mutable water sign that integrates influences from each of the eleven signs that precede it. Bringing a focus on oneness, Pisces encourages you to understand nuance, blending spirituality and practicality to increase empathy, healing capacities, and intuitive knowing. Under a Pisces moon, you may be drawn toward nonverbal, artistic pursuits. Pay attention to boundaries to avoid over-giving. Stay open to psychic channels, practice meditation, listen to music, or watch an inspiring movie.

New Moon in Pisces: This is a great time to set intentions to amplify your psychic capacity. Keep in mind, though, that while all new moons represent a new beginning, a new moon in Pisces simultaneously signifies a completion of the astrological year. As you eagerly move in the direction of what you most desire, focus on healing and forgiveness.

Full Moon in Pisces: This intuitive full moon activates the Pisces-Virgo axis. Honor your intuition. Forgiveness is cosmic medicine now, as is sadness, vulnerability, and honesty about your fears. You are invited to lean into the arts and spiritual exploration in order to bring your dreams into reality and process your emotions. Stay mindful of feeling like a victim, engaging in escapism, and/or resorting to addiction.

Emotional Self-Care as a Foundation for Self-Worth

When I first met Claire, she was a stay-at-home mother of three, who dreamed of starting her own business. Each time she'd tried to start one, she'd abandoned the effort, feeling deep discomfort around prioritizing herself over her family's needs. But Claire, a white woman living in a rural community, yearned to contribute to her family's income and disrupt the patterns of self-abnegation that undermined her desire for growth. However, not earning money, she felt, was proof she didn't deserve to take up physical space in her home or energetic space in her calendar. She was in a vicious cycle.

As we began working together to unlock her cosmic health, Claire connected to her deep desire to create an area in her house where she could work on her new business. One day she bought an old side table at a garage sale, grabbed a folding chair, and placed them in a corner in her house. That tiny space was her first "home office"—and the beginning of the life she'd dreamed of living.

As she tuned in to her deeper needs, she also realized that she had been prioritizing her family's needs over her own self-care as a way to avoid her fear. By syncing her self-care to lunar cycles, she was able to add herself to her list of priorities. As her self-care began to mirror and support her deeper emotional needs, her business began to grow and, with it, her need for more space. First reclaiming an unused room in her house, then a neighbor's shed, and finally relocating to a leased office space, Claire built a name for herself as a consultant.

Doing this wasn't easy. Claire had to continually face emotions that felt tricky and overwhelming—scary, even—especially when they surged with intensity. Claire experienced this repeatedly as she took up space in her own home. The mere thought of repainting a wall in her home office felt overwhelming at first. She didn't feel she was "allowed" to make that kind of mark on a room. Instead of giving in to her fear, however, she listened to her desire. Although still afraid, she continued to take action, which enabled her to grow and evolve to where she is now—finding ownership in her home and her life, and thriving as a result. Claire tapped into her cosmic health, and it has since transformed her emotional, spiritual, physical, and financial health.

Now she not only has grown her business substantially but also pays more attention to her physical body, which she sees as critical to her continued flourishing as a business owner, and as a wife and mom. Tuned into her monthly rhythms, she can now anticipate when she needs extra sleep, which has helped her optimize her energy and focus all month long. She also moves her body more, incorporating more yoga and running into her schedule. She feels better—more energized and happier—than she has in a very long time.

All of these changes—the growth of her business, the massive transformation in her self-esteem, improvements in her health and self-care—came from tending to her emotions.

I love how Claire continued to use the moon to expand and deepen her own awareness. In addition to optimizing sleep and movement to complement her nutrition, her new sense of emotional well-being awakened her desire to be of service in even bigger ways. Once her self-confidence grew, she connected to a deeper yearning to work in environmental activism within her local community. Her work as an activist is challenging, especially since she has to stand up to people in power. But, she's learned how to take bigger risks and live with more bravery.

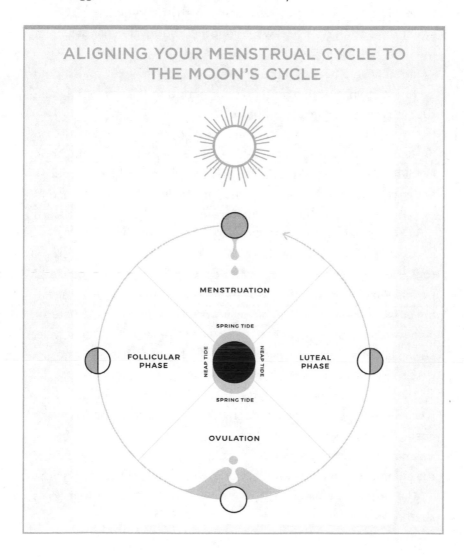

ALIGNING YOUR MENSTRUAL CYCLE TO THE MOON'S CYCLE

MENSTRUATION

SPRING TIDE

NEAP TIDE

FOLLICULAR PHASE

NEAP TIDE

LUTEAL PHASE

SPRING TIDE

OVULATION

Syncing your menstrual cycle with the moon means bleeding with the new moon and ovulating with the full moon. Before electricity, history suggests that this happened regularly. So achieving this in the age of technology feels like an awesome intersection of power.

But I want you to know that matching these two cycles is not necessary. Perhaps even contraindicated for achieving your health goals.

Here's why: If you menstruate, maintaining a healthy cycle needs to be your number-one priority. And a healthy cycle is approximately twenty-one to thirty-five days long with the sweet spot being twenty-five to thirty-five days in length.[5] Your cycle changes all of the time, but the moon's cycle never does.

If you have a healthy, regular menstrual cycle, your goal should be to maintain it. Trying to align your period to the moon may disrupt it, creating unnecessary harm.

If you don't have a healthy menstrual cycle, set your sights on healing this first. Doing so will take work, and syncing with the moon is not the first step. Holistically healing your menstrual cycle requires eating a blood-sugar balancing diet, optimizing your digestion, and repairing your hypothalamic-pituitary-adrenal (HPA) axis. (To learn more, check out Nicole Jardim's book *Fix Your Period*.)

If you don't menstruate due to a hysterectomy or being postpartum, if you suffer from amenorrhea or irregular periods because of perimenopause or any other issue that dysregulates your period, if you are prepubescent, if you identify as a woman but don't menstruate, or if you are nonbinary and want to work with the energetics of this cycle, keying into the moon's cadence will help you to access this rhythm. It's precisely what I've done for over two decades, and it works like magic!

The new moon represents the menstruating phase of the cycle, while the waxing phase of the moon mirrors the follicular phase, which spans the days between the start of a period and ovulation. The full moon emulates the energy of ovulation. Finally, the waning portion of the moon's cycle mimics the luteal, or premenstrual, phase of the cycle.

The process of syncing your hormonal rhythm with the moon's rhythm is known as "phase shifting." This means altering your behaviors, as well as your environment, to match the environmental cues and light stimulus of the cycle of the moon.[6]

To entrain your menstrual cycle to match the moon's rhythm requires you to honor the darkness associated with the moon. That requires you to avoid light at night during the period between the waning crescent moon through the first two days after the new moon. No computers or TV after dinner. As the moon waxes, begin to incrementally expose yourself to more light each night. At the full moon, you really want to be in light all night, even as you sleep. Then reverse the process as the moon wanes.

Here are some tips to get you started:

1. Begin by simultaneously tracking your menstrual cycle and the lunar cycle, first by noticing where you are in your menstrual cycle at the time of the new moon. Are you bleeding? Ovulating? Are you between your period and ovulation (the follicular phase)? Or are you between ovulation and your period (the luteal phase)? If the new moon falls when you are at the earliest part of your period, you will likely ovulate close to the full moon. If the new moon falls when you are ovulating, you are at the opposite, which offers a potent intersection of power too. You may also be in the follicular or luteal phase at the new moon. Log both cycles, trusting that wherever you are is perfect.

2. Once you get a sense of where you are in your cycle at the time of the new moon, you can begin to consciously work with the lunar and menstrual rhythms. The new moon is a more internal, intention-setting time, while ovulation, hormonally speaking, is a more energized time of the month. However, it's important to honor your body's needs first and then layer in the lunar rhythm from there.

3. Starting on a new moon, set your intention to harmonize your body's rhythm with the lunar rhythm. For one whole cycle, track the moon daily, getting outside to see the moon and acknowledge its changes.

4. During the moon's new, waxing crescent, and waxing quarter phases, as well as the waning quarter and waning crescent phases, make sure you shut down your technology early, employ a soothing nighttime ritual, and focus on sleep hygiene and rest. Draw your blinds and sleep in a pitch-black room. Between the waxing gibbous and waning gibbous phases, allow yourself extra exposure to the moon's light. Aligning with the moon's light, as opposed to artificial light, gives your biology the chance to sync with the moon's cadence.

5. Here's where this becomes a bit dangerous to your body. During the waxing gibbous, full, and waning gibbous phases, you actually want to expose yourself to more light at night. You can do this by keeping the blinds open so moonlight infiltrates your room or sleeping with a light on—approximately 100-watt voltage—for three nights. Please note, using light at night with the intention of changing your hormonal rhythm will likely disrupt your sleep and can unnecessarily dysregulate your hormonal cycle.

To learn even more about the lunar phases and the menstrual cycle, download the free companion *Cosmic Health* ebook at JenniferRacioppi.com/resources. Also, check out Kate Northrup's OriginCollective.com.

Magic is a way of living. If one has done one's best to steer the chariot, and one then notices that a greater other is actually steering it, then magical operations have taken place. One cannot say what the effect of magic will be, since no one can know in advance because the magical is lawless, which occurs without rules and by chance, so to speak.

—C. G. JUNG, FROM *THE RED BOOK*

Building an Altar: Create the Conditions for Success

An altar can be set up in a specific spot in your home or office and sanctified as a special place to commune with the divine. I advise experimenting with how you set it up. Consider placing sacred objects on your altar that represent each of the elements in the zodiac. Here are some suggestions:

Air: An inspiring image

Fire: A candle

Water: A bowl of water

Earth: A small plant

When crafting an altar, it's important to think about your own ancestry and heritage, your spiritual beliefs. What can you put on it that's reflective of you? Maybe you want a picture of you as a child and pictures of loved ones. Perhaps there are other sacred items that remind you of your heritage, your dreams, and your goals. Make a list. These objects should help you feel a direct connection to the divine. Treat gathering items and setting up your altar like a scavenger hunt. Let synchronicity support you, and see what comes up. Give yourself a few days to gather your items, and when you are ready, create your altar.

Remember, this work is about accessing your truth, not following someone else's rules. Your altar is your sacred space, and it needs to represent you, and your ancestry. It's a place to honor your devotional practice. As you move through the book, you will find that the ritual practices build off one another. Go at your own pace.

Identifying Your Vision

Take some time and consider your vision for your healing journey; get crystal clear on what you wish to create. It's essential to begin to visualize, see, dream, and imagine the healing you wish to conjure. Let yourself play, daydream, fantasize. Think outside the box. Then write down your vision. Dwell on this, allowing it to come to life inside you. Read it out loud. You may notice that your vision evokes even more emotion when spoken; that feeling is essential to the act of co-creating.

Then, ask yourself this: *What becomes possible for me if I realize this life vision?* Journal your answers. When you are done, read what you wrote out loud to yourself.

Now ponder this question: *What is holding me back from realizing this vision?* Take time and journal your answers.

Finally, commit to realizing change in your life. Write out your commitment and place it on your altar. Each time you go to your altar, read it out loud.

Now that we've looked at how the moon can affect our experience, we'll look next at our relationship to the sun, which also plays a critical role in our health.

CHAPTER 4

Living in Sync with Solar Cycles

One day in the Vale of Nysa, Persephone, daughter of Demeter (goddess of agriculture) and Zeus (chief god), was picking flowers by a stream when Zeus's brother Hades (king of the underworld) seized her and took her to the underworld. Upon learning of the abduction, Demeter was so overcome by grief that the flowers and crops ceased to grow. For an entire year, a great famine befell Earth as Demeter's sorrow overpowered her.

Zeus eventually intervened, and Hades agreed to return Persephone to her mother. Before releasing her, however, Hades tricked Persephone into eating a pomegranate seed, food of the dead. From that point on, Persephone was compelled to live a portion of each year in the underworld with Hades.

As the myth goes, each time Persephone is absent, Demeter descends once again into her grief, causing flowers and crops to die, creating what we now know as autumn and winter. Each time Persephone returns to her mother, the Earth can once again blossom, thus allowing for spring and summer.

Seasonal living is as ancient as Earth itself. It nourishes us, supports our needs, and awakens our power to transform. We'll begin to synchronize ourselves with this seasonality, which is inherent in the practice of astrology, by attuning ourselves and our health to the cycles of the sun.

The Sun, the Seasons, and Our Health

As we navigate the four seasons, we simultaneously experience the dance between differing periods of sunlight and darkness, day and night. This is especially significant because sunlight plays a vital role in our health and healing.

This is why many of us experience seasonal mood swings during the shorter days of fall and winter, when our circadian rhythm is thrown off. Less light during the day has been linked to lower production of serotonin, the neurotransmitter that influences feelings of well-being and happiness.[1]

Low serotonin can lead to depression and anxiety—the "winter blues." It can also cause high-carb comfort-food cravings, since eating carbohydrates temporarily increases serotonin levels.[2] Changing light levels also affect melatonin production in the brain.[3] As the body is exposed to fewer hours of sunlight during shorter winter days, it produces more melatonin, making us feel sleepier.

Instead of pushing back against seasonal, sunlight-related changes in energy, we can respect the body's need for sunlight while also embracing the various seasonal shifts as essential to our growth.

Harnessing the Healing Power of Sunshine

I was twenty years old when I began to understand how profoundly sunlight affected me, both physically and emotionally. Ready to begin anew, I felt a deep yearning to live somewhere else—*without* the stigma of who I once was and *away* from the people who knew me through cancer. In true natal-sun-in-Gemini fashion, I was *out*. With one backpack and very little money, I boarded a plane to San Diego, where my then-boyfriend was living.

Although still in a fragile post-cancer/post-menopausal state, I wasn't kidding myself. It was a big move, and leaving home meant becoming radically self-reliant, not just personally but financially too. What I didn't realize when I walked onto that cross-country flight was that San Diego would respond to my bold risk-taking by giving me an extended and deeply nourishing solar hug.

Almost immediately, San Diego felt like a warm blanket of serenity. I quickly settled into a routine — at least, as much of a routine as a twenty-year-old food server who was establishing residency in California while waiting to return to college full-time could manage. Fairly quickly, my body calmed as my levels of cortisol, the "stress hormone," recalibrated to healthier levels. I frequently took long walks on the beach — and spent as much time as I could outside, near the ocean.

A couple of months into living in my new home, something miraculous happened. I began to sleep at night — as in, I'd close my eyes and just, well, sleep. Since early childhood sleep had felt like an enemy with a single purpose: to haunt me. Keeping me up when I should be dreaming peacefully, robbing me of much-needed energy and focus each day, nonsensical sleep patterns had tortured me for years.

Living a quiet life in sun-drenched San Diego healed my circadian rhythm, and my energy and my mental/emotional state improved dramatically. I now knew what it felt like to wake up rejuvenated. At long last I had energy, concentration, and focus. I could show up each day and do my job seamlessly, which also meant I could continue to afford to live there.

Finally reconciled with my circadian rhythm, I found that so much seemed possible — in my life as well as my health and happiness. It also proved to be a gateway to seasonal catharsis, which, as we'll discuss next, is a critical element of cyclical, seasonal living, and the even deeper healing it provides.

SUNLIGHT, THE BODY, AND OUR HEALTH

When people are exposed to the sunrise, they experience a 50 percent drop in mood disorders.[4] Bright light in the morning lowers morning melatonin levels and increases cortisol—exactly what you want to have happen so you awaken refreshed.[5] A more regular ebb and flow of these two hormones may be why, according to a study, people who get bright morning light report fewer sleep disturbances.[6] Plus, morning light increases insulin sensitivity, meaning you'll need less insulin to keep your blood sugar levels balanced and you'll lower your risk for many diseases, including diabetes.[7]

Seasons: An Invitation to Transform

Each season offers us an opportunity for catharsis. The term itself comes from the Greek word *katharsis*, meaning "purification" or "cleansing." It relates to the release of emotions in a therapeutic way. Catharsis is an opportunity to release. That's what autumn provides: an opportunity to shed what is no longer serving us. Winter allows us to lie fallow, listen, and plant seeds for what we wish to cultivate next. Early spring is a time of hunger, when the seeds we planted in winter haven't yet germinated. By summer, we revel in the bounty and abundant sunshine. This is the essence of our seasonal rhythm.

Inherent in the solar cycles of the four seasons is transformation in our emotions. This is how we access the power of cyclical living. To live seasonally means to embrace the cathartic gifts that the changes in length of day and weather provide. It's not always easy to let go of what we know and believe. The resistance we feel around this process of shedding contributes to the seasonal "blues" many of us experience.

While it's natural to feel resistance around change, this discomfort is baked into transformation. Change, however unsettling, offers us an opportunity for growth, which then leads us toward restoration and renewal. Leaning into these cycles of change, syncing our health journey to the seasons, and adapting our self-care accordingly are central to optimizing our health, which acts as a foundation for flourishing in all parts of our lives.

I connected with this deeper yearning for seasonal catharsis after many months in San Diego. The stasis and balance I'd initially found there led me to crave change and growth. I longed to return to a more pronounced cyclical modulation provided by all four seasons. As nourishing as the sunshine had felt, ultimately I missed the deep catharsis that autumn and winter, with their shorter days and colder temperatures, enable. That's not to say you can't live seasonally when it's temperate year-round. You can. The days are still shorter in the winter and longer in the summer. You are still experiencing the magic of Earth revolving around the sun. I just craved a more substantial experience of winter, and—dare I even say it?—rain!

These seasonal cycles of change and transformation have been happening for billions of years. Even when we "hate" autumn and winter, as I once thought I did, we eventually discover that these cycles are the essential link between our outer and inner worlds.

LIVING IN SYNC WITH THE SUN

As Earth makes its way around the sun, we experience several phenomena that play important roles in our health journey: four distinct seasons, four cross-quarter days (the halfway point of each season), and the sun's apparent ongoing transit through the twelve zodiac signs.

As we delve deeper into syncing our lives to the solar cycles, keep in mind that your experience of the seasons will depend on where you live. Certain parts of the world have more distinct seasons than others. Climate change is altering weather patterns worldwide too. Also, the Southern Hemisphere experiences seasons at opposite times of the year from the Northern Hemisphere (summer in the Northern Hemisphere is winter in the Southern Hemisphere, and vice versa).

Let's look first at the basic anatomy of a complete sun cycle and then walk through an astrological year, season by season, and one zodiac sign at a time, to get a clearer sense of how this all plays out.

The Anatomy of a Complete Solar Cycle

At the time of a *solstice*—which comes from Latin *sol* ("sun") combined with *sistere* ("to stand still" or "to stop")—the sun, on the ecliptic, reaches its maximum distance from the celestial equator. When it is at its most northerly position (the Tropic of Cancer) we have the June solstice; at its most southerly position (the Tropic of Capricorn) is the December solstice. On the June solstice, the sun is at zero degrees of Cancer, and on the December solstice, zero degrees of Capricorn.

Tropikós, in ancient Greek, means "a turn." That's exactly what the sun appears to do at the time of the solstice: stop, for roughly three days, and then turn around.

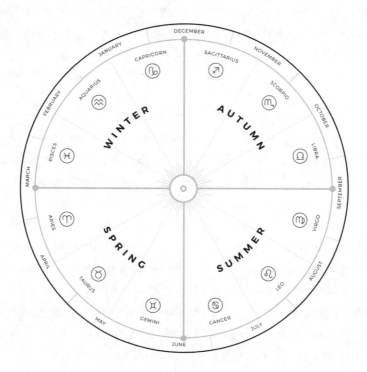

An *equinox*, which is roughly translated from Latin as "equal night," occurs when the sun, on the ecliptic, crosses the celestial equator. On the March equinox, the sun is at zero degrees of Aries, and at the September equinox, zero degrees of Libra.[8]

WHY THE SOUTHERN AND NORTHERN HEMISPHERES HAVE OPPOSITE SEASONS

As we discussed in chapter 2, the tropical zodiac is based on the cardinal directions that form at the solstice and equinox points. The planes of rotation created by the celestial equator (Earth's equator projected into space) and the ecliptic (the sun's apparent path around the Earth) intersect at the equinoxes and have their greatest declination at the time of the solstices.

Earth's 23.4° axial tilt, also known as the obliquity of the ecliptic, is responsible for the seasons. It is why each hemisphere is exposed to more or less sun at certain times of the year. It's also why the Northern and Southern hemispheres experience opposite seasons. But that doesn't mean they experience different zodiac signs. The sun is in the same zodiac sign for the entire world at the same time.

I spoke with Gemini Brett when writing this book, and he said, "The tropical zodiac, like so many shamanic traditions, aligns with the energies of the cardinal directions. The tropical zodiac is indeed seasonal as it is often presented, but tropical astrologers rarely acknowledge seasonal opposition between Earth's hemispheres. The key is that the north is north from everywhere on Earth."

While this chapter focuses on the zodiac from the Northern Hemisphere perspective, know this: the tropical zodiac is seasonal, but the seasons don't define the zodiac signs. Our experience of the annual seasonal rhythm will be different from those who live in the Southern Hemisphere, but the essence of the sign remains the same. To learn more about astronomy for astrology, check out GeminiBrett.com.

The Sun and the Twelve Signs of the Zodiac

Each season encompasses three zodiac signs, and as a reminder, the signs within each season always proceed in this order: a *cardinal* sign initiates the season, a *fixed* sign stabilizes the season, and a *mutable* sign prepares us for the coming change of season.

Solar Cycle Overview (Northern Hemisphere)

Note: The exact days when the sun enters a new sign vary from year to year. Please check your calendar for the most accurate dates.

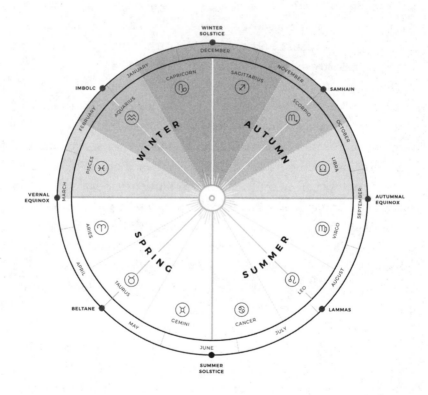

Vernal equinox: March 21
  Aries (cardinal fire)
  Taurus (fixed earth)
Beltane, cross-quarter marker: May 1
  Gemini (mutable air)
Summer solstice: June 21
  Cancer (cardinal water)
  Leo (fixed fire)
Lammas, cross-quarter marker: August 1
  Virgo (mutable earth)
Autumnal equinox: September 21
  Libra (cardinal air)
  Scorpio (fixed water)
Samhain, cross-quarter marker: November 1
  Sagittarius (mutable fire)
Winter solstice: December 21
  Capricorn (cardinal earth)
  Aquarius (fixed air)
Imbolc, cross-quarter marker: February 1
  Pisces (mutable water)

WHAT ARE THE CROSS-QUARTER DAYS?

While the solstices and equinoxes divide the year into four seasons, each season is divided by a cross-quarter day, which is always in a fixed sign and signifies the halfway point between a solstice and an equinox.

Beltane initiates us into the season of growth. Readying yourself for a cycle of expansion will serve your health during this period. Spending time outdoors, eating fresh food, and getting plenty of exercise allow you to make the most of the spring season. This day celebrates fertility.

Lammas welcomes us into the season of harvest. The abundance of summer must now be cultivated. It's especially important to be eating lots of fresh, local foods at this time, as well as prioritizing joy and pleasure.

Samhain beckons us inward. This is one of the most sacred times of year, when we commune with darkness and our inner wisdom. The days become shorter, so prioritizing sleep becomes very important. Additionally, transitioning your diet from the light, bright foods of late summer and early fall to the richer foods of winter serves you well now.

Imbolc symbolizes the rebirth of hope. We celebrate the anticipated return of light and growth while knowing that a significant amount of darkness remains. This is a time of year to bring your focus to your spiritual development. Staying devoted to the light within helps you nourish and nurture your wisdom.

The Astrological Seasons and Zodiacal Living

Next we'll move through each of the zodiac signs as they relate to the seasons. Keep in mind, the guidance provided in this chapter is to help you adjust your self-care to the seasonality of the sign the sun travels through, so it applies to all, regardless of our personal astrology charts.

The Zodiac Signs of Spring

As we saw in chapter 2, the astrological year begins with Aries, which marks the start of spring in the Northern Hemisphere. Spring encompasses **Aries** (cardinal fire), **Taurus** (fixed earth), and **Gemini** (mutable air).

ADAPTING SELF-CARE IN SPRING

People tend to think of spring as lush, blooming, and full of life, but really, in early spring, particularly in the Northern Hemisphere, nothing is ready for harvest yet. While we feel the promise of the abundance to come, it isn't yet available. This is a time of emergence, in the natural world and inside the self, a time to initiate new beginnings based on the wisdom we gained during the autumn and winter.

The roots we set down now will carry us through the year ahead. The March equinox is the astrological new year, making spring a powerful time to match movement with intention, create an altar, or craft personal and professional goals.

To balance the transition from late winter into early spring, support your liver. Minimize complex carbohydrates, reduce your consumption of sugar, take a high-quality multivitamin, eat a blood-sugar balanced diet with lots of leafy greens and high-quality proteins, and drink plenty of water. Prioritize sweating.

In addition to this "decluttering" of the physical body, it's a good time to declutter your physical environment with a spring clean and begin anew.

♈ Aries

This cardinal fire sign marks the start of the astrological year. It represents the beginning.

Zero degrees Aries is the vernal equinox in the Northern Hemisphere and the autumnal equinox in the Southern Hemisphere.

Aries activates ambition, drive, passion, determination, and action. It rules the head, and is an invitation to embrace sovereignty and independence, renew your energy, and reclaim your ambition. Aries's influence brings a sense of urgency, a desire to make space, start anew, and powerfully eliminate that which you no longer need.

Patience can be in short supply at this time. Use this energy wisely—wake up early to soak in the morning sunlight; engage in physical movement that makes you sweat. On an emotional level, since this time correlates with anger and impatience, it's important to cathartically release emotions in healthy ways—for example, through exercise, expressive writing/arts, activism, or therapy.

♉ *Taurus*

This fixed earth sign plants us firmly in the *center* of the season.

Taurus season awakens desires for sensuality, sexual pleasure, and physical embodiment. Ruled by Venus, the planet of love and beauty, Taurus is about nurturing your erotic nature, and committing to growth. As a time ruled by a fixed earth sign, Taurus season is also a time to leverage stability in order to catapult your sense of personal agency. When possible, put your bare feet on the ground and connect to the earth.

Since Taurus rules the throat, try singing or chanting. Doing so stimulates the diaphragm, lengthening your breath and potentially even releasing tension in the pelvic floor. Another way to amplify the connection between your voice and body is to speak positive affirmations out loud in front of a mirror. Loving your body, exactly as it is today, is a part of health.

♊ *Gemini*

Gemini is the first mutable sign of the zodiac and bridges seasons.

Mercury, the messenger, rules Gemini. Mercury asks us to assimilate knowledge by forging connections that previously didn't exist. Learning new things through travel, writing, and socializing are especially useful during this time of year.

Gemini rules your shoulders, arms, and hands, making this a time of dexterity. But on the downside, it can also be a season of haste. Socializing can quickly give way to superficial interactions—watch out for this tendency. When possible, keep 20 percent of your calendar free of commitments. Being overscheduled at this time is likely but can also increase nervousness, anxiety, and restlessness. To offset these tendencies, eat healthily and practice mindfulness. Activities like forest bathing, or *shinrin-yoku*, the Japanese practice of immersing yourself in nature for better mental and physical health, are beneficial now. They provide grounding and balance the fast-paced, mutable air energy of Gemini.

The Zodiac Signs of Summer

This is the second season of the astrological year—summer in the Northern Hemisphere—and it encompasses **Cancer** (cardinal water), **Leo** (fixed fire), and **Virgo** (mutable earth).

ADAPTING SELF-CARE IN SUMMER

Welcome to the season of light. With increased sunlight exposure, the body's serotonin levels are naturally higher, making summer a joyful season. It invites you to wake up earlier, go to bed later, expand your heart, and engage in laughter so strong it makes your belly hurt.

Summer is a season of play, but with so many social activities it can also lead to burnout, especially if mindful self-care isn't employed. Drink lots of water, be aware of people-pleasing tendencies, and avoid getting overly busy. Swimming in lakes, streams, ponds, oceans, and pools not only cools you down but nourishes your yin energy too.

Summer-related imbalances include sunburn, hot flashes, exhaustion, acne, and digestive issues. Emotionally, excess heat can manifest as anger, jealousy, or impatience. To counteract this, stay mindful of what you do midday. When possible, eat lots of locally grown foods, especially fruits and vegetables. With plenty of opportunities for outdoor activity, the fresh air and sunlight (hello, vitamin D!) also deliver important bacteria that nourish your gut microbiome.

♋ Cancer

This cardinal water sign begins the second season of the astrological year.

Ruled by the moon, Cancer season requires a courageous commitment to love—to love those we nurture and those who nurture us. Simultaneously, we are asked to understand the cavernous nature of our emotional needs, and to meet more of them through radical self-care. This is a time to deepen roots, including with family, and gain a more profound understanding of the divine feminine.

Honor your ancestors, the difficulties they faced and the legacy they left, by remembering them. Tell their stories. If your family story affects you adversely, take time to gently feel this. What's there for you to heal?

The body parts associated with nurturing—the chest and breast—are highlighted now. The modern world is full of xenoestrogens, synthetic chemicals that mimic the effects of estrogen. This can lead to estrogen dominance, when the body has excess estrogen and/or when estrogen levels are too high in relation to progesterone levels. Cancer season offers the opportunity to indulge in an abundance of locally grown and detoxifying foods, which support a healthy metabolism and the elimination of excess estrogen. By keeping your bowels regular and healthy, being sure to sweat daily, and tending to your liver by eating lots of leafy greens plus limiting alcohol and sugar, you help your body balance its hormones naturally. Doing so is protective of the breasts.

♌ Leo

This fixed fire sign marks the *center* of the second season of the astrological year.

To encompass Leo energy, you need to metaphorically live from your center—the heart. That means avidly pursuing what you love while also practicing unconditional self-love. Loving yourself feels easy when you're the bright light you want yourself to be; self-love feels harder when you face the shadows that make us all human. By integrating your internal light and darkness, including the lessons each has to offer, you can become the powerful, sovereign leader you are meant to be. Practices like visualization, meditation, dance, and singing provide a healing bridge between the "work" associated with self-love and the joy it brings.

During Leo season, take time to honor your inner child, bravely expressing yourself with authenticity and originality. Stay openhearted and bring your commitment—and genuine excitement—to bear every day. This is when you should play like your heart depends on it.

Leo rules the upper back and heart. Paradoxically, a strong core helps you to stand tall, like a lion. Pilates is a low-impact exercise system that lengthens the torso, strengthens the core, and helps to develop self-awareness. If this practice is new to you, try out a mat Pilates class. You can find one online!

As you step into your sovereignty, trust your body to guide your food choices by embracing intuitive eating.

♍ Virgo

This mutable earth sign prepares you to leave behind the current season and ready yourself for what's ahead.

Virgo marks a turning point. This is a time of year to clear out the proverbial old, reduce indulgences, and choose nourishment. If Leo season is a time to discover your "yes," Virgo season is a time to honor your "no." Check in with your body and ask yourself which types of exercise, food, people, and experiences are aligned with your highest purpose. Streamline and stay in service to what matters most as you move into the coming season.

Virgo season is also a call for devotion to purpose. It asks you to assimilate your lessons and focus on what matters most to you. I lovingly refer to Virgo as the protector of purity. This season asks you to protect what is most meaningful.

At this time of year, focus too on your digestion. To support your body's ability to absorb nutrients and eliminate toxins, take extra care to chew your food. Digestion starts in your mouth. Eat mindfully and slowly when you can, tasting and enjoying your food.

NAVIGATING THE "END OF SUMMER FUNK"

Does the approaching end of summer get to you around this time each year? It makes sense. Life has been bursting all around you for months, pulling your attention outward. Just as you adjust to this state of being, it's time for change yet again. It's natural to feel some resistance. In my younger years, that opposition meant heading face first into the "end of summer funk."

What I've learned through years of personal development is that sadness at this seasonal turning point usually comes because of a failure to tend to the inner world. Meditation went out the window in early spring. Solo activities disappeared soon afterward. And nourishing the body with nutrient-rich foods? That hasn't happened since sometime in June.

All the fun of the outer world has pulled your attention away from your connection to self—the part of you that's grounded, nurturing, and can find appreciation in the flow of Earth's cycles. With the season beginning to shift, it's the perfect time to repair that connection. Return home to yourself and reestablish self-care routines.

The Zodiac Signs of Autumn

This third season of the astrological year—autumn in the Northern Hemisphere—encompasses **Libra** (cardinal air), **Scorpio** (fixed water), and **Sagittarius** (mutable fire).

ADAPTING SELF-CARE IN AUTUMN

The autumnal, or September, equinox brings an equal balance between day and night. Occurring in the middle of harvest season, the darker and shorter days ahead require that we adapt to decreased sunlight.

The winds of change provide more movement around us — in the trees and throughout the natural world — and also within ourselves. Yet with the unpredictability of climate change, in the modern age autumn also brings unstable weather patterns, especially during hurricane season, when the winds blow too strongly. Fall asks us to be ready for anything, which is why it's important to enter this season mindfully.

Decreased sunlight reduces serotonin levels, which can introduce seasonal affective disorder. At this time we may experience melancholy or feel flighty, restless, or anxious. Prioritize skin care since your skin may feel dry. Sesame oil is a great body moisturizer, and hydrating face masks are helpful at night. Castor oil foot massages are especially healing too (add a dram of sandalwood essential oil for extra grounding).

Nourish your digestion at this time of year too, as the change in weather and exposure to sun can slow down your metabolism.

During this time of waning light, also process your emotions. In Chinese medicine autumn is the season of sadness, grief, and worry, and is connected to the lungs. Cathartic activities like art, music, dancing, writing, therapy, yoga, and even going to the theater are seasonally applicable.

♎ Libra

This cardinal air sign kicks off the third season of the astrological year.

Since Libra brings opposites together, which we witness in the natural world via the equinox, Libra season bodes well for socializing. At this time we are asked to come into a right relationship with our values and strive for equanimity, balance, and justice. Libra also represents fashion, inspiring us to make wardrobe changes or home decoration adjustments and indulge our creativity.

Being mindful of falling into codependent dynamics is also a priority now. Bending over backwards to please others may make you susceptible to lower back pain. Overexertion can also lead to adrenal imbalances. This is the time to practice yin yoga poses that work on the kidney meridian—sphinx, butterfly, or reclining twist poses are some to try.

The underlying lesson of Libra is to stay in alignment with your truth while also tuning in to others.

♏ *Scorpio*

This fixed water sign places us in the *center* of the season.

Co-ruled by Pluto and Mars, Scorpio season awakens us to our sexuality and asks us to lean into the healing power of orgasm. Whereas Libra is about recalibration and equilibrium, Scorpio season is a time of intimacy, connection with our innermost needs, and introspection. Let's face it, the modern world leaves little time for this, especially with the holiday season quickly approaching. Give yourself the quiet time you crave to assess the lessons of transformation as you step into a more evolved version of your authentic self.

Long-buried feelings of shame may also bubble up to the surface. By bringing the darkness to light, you create opportunities for healing. Stay mindful of addictions and other escapist outlets.

Since Scorpio relates to your sexual health, nourishing and nurturing your sexuality goes a long way now. Explore your sexuality either with a partner or through masturbation; maybe even buy yourself a new toy. If sex is painful for you physically, consider pelvic floor physical therapy. If you have a history of sexual trauma, starting traditional therapy or trauma therapy at this time of year bodes well.

↗ *Sagittarius*

This mutable fire sign spans the gap between seasons, creating a bold, blunt, adventurous mood.

You've done the internal, uncomfortable deep dive during Scorpio season, so now you can shake off those revelations and live in the present moment. Ruled by Jupiter, the planet of good luck and blessings, Sagittarius brings you jovial, extroverted energy that encourages you to follow your joy.

It also offers you a time of growth. However, if left unchecked, this season can lead to excess and overindulgence. Emotionally and spiritually, this is a time to revel in gratitude, abundance, and optimism. But do stay mindful of overindulgence, a hallmark of this time of year. Amidst the holiday frenzy, it's easy to feel stressed and sad. Remember, emotions guide you to pay attention to your inner needs.

Sagittarius rules the hips, a part of the body often said to hold emotions. With the new year and solstice just ahead, spend time contemplating the year that's soon to end. What did you learn? What are you celebrating? What are you grieving? Name the emotions you are experiencing. Then massage your hips with a body lotion or oil. As you do, let yourself feel what's coming up for you.

The Zodiac Signs of Winter

This fourth and final season of the astrological year—winter in the Northern Hemisphere—encompasses **Capricorn** (cardinal earth), **Aquarius** (fixed air), and **Pisces** (mutable water).

> ## ADAPTING SELF-CARE IN WINTER
>
> This is the time to turn inward, rest, recuperate, and listen to your inner voice. Spend time cultivating meaningful relationships and engaging with purpose.

The lack of sunlight means decreased serotonin levels in the body, making this feel like a season of retreat. Remember, this is part of the natural cycle of catharsis. We have to shed and release in order to grow. We have to allow for death in order to usher in rebirth. If fear comes up at this time of year, lean in and learn. How can you feel your pain without becoming your pain?

Winter is a season of yin restoration, a time when nature goes dormant, yet underneath, the raw power required to grow and evolve remains strong, working hard beneath the surface to rejuvenate itself. While this can be a time for extended focus on work, do also take time to nourish yourself from the inside out. The long nights provide ample opportunity for restorative sleep and rest.

♑ Capricorn

A cardinal earth sign, Capricorn initiates the fourth and final season of the astrological year.

Ruled by Saturn, Capricorn season asks you to develop a routine that will keep you grounded and focused on moving toward your purpose. Turn toward what you've learned in the previous season and use it to build a solid base. Capricorn is associated with the knees and bones, which literally create our frame and hold us upright. Stretching and yoga are particularly powerful movements to engage in at this time of year. If you lack the mobility required for this, use your breath to connect with your bones.

Since Capricorn is both cardinal and earth, to reach your highest potential, embrace the paradox of practical wisdom. Now is the time to achieve by mastering the less flashy elements of life—routine, habits, and structure. Anything is attainable with time, patience, and the proper inner resources. It's winter, a time of rest, but also the new year, a time of ambition. Learning how to nourish yourself without overextending becomes critical now. At the same time, channeling your energy on behalf of your most important goals proves prudent during this season.

♒ *Aquarius*

A fixed air sign, Aquarius falls in the *center* of the season.

Co-ruled by Saturn and Uranus, Aquarius brings the disruptive innovation that comes from forced reflection and the slower pace that supports the birthing of new ideas. Aquarius season invites quick thinking. It's a time to tune in to the collective energy of growth and stimulation. To support this, you are well advised to develop a morning routine, which will help you feel grounded and connected with your inner emotional world first and foremost, before you take on the outer world.

Aquarius rules the ankles, helping you to stay balanced as you step into the future. The key to health is being able to individuate and separate. To that end, you may be driven to find community and become part of a crowd—just not the mainstream crowd. Instead, this is the time to focus on finding *your* people.

♓ *Pisces*

As the last sign of the zodiac, and mutable water, this season marks the end of the astrological calendar.

The most spiritually compounded sign of the zodiac, Pisces understands oneness, so empathizing with others and anticipating their needs comes easily now. This time is about mystical attunement. You also gain a strong understanding of nuance, which asks you to blend your spirituality with practicality. However, beware of overgiving, as it's all too easy to lose yourself if you don't work on boundaries now.

Another way to transcend the mundane is through dreams. Co-ruled by imaginative Neptune and beneficent Jupiter, Pisces provides support for your visions: they are potent and possible now. Think of artistic pursuits as a way to give yourself a much-needed time-out from physical reality—dance, paint, or draw your way back to emotional equilibrium.

This is a time to take extra care of your feet (your grounding force in life), as well as the immune system, especially the lymphatic system. Separating from your surroundings and creating space for yourself is recommended. Daily meditation can be especially healing now.

Ritual: Aligning with Your Wisdom

This ritual is best done after reading this chapter or whenever you need to access your wisdom. You will need a journal and a pen.

Begin by centering with a brief meditation.

Honor your breath. Check in with your mind. Do you feel clear and focused, or scattered and anxious? Breathe into whatever it is, with acceptance, compassion, and love.

Honor your spirit. How courageous do you feel? What's inspiring you now? How can you feel even more inspired and courageous today? Take a moment to feel this. When you're ready, move to the next direction.

Honor your intuition. Check in with your higher self. How do you feel today? What is your intuition asking you to acknowledge? What's coming up for you emotionally? Get quiet and hear what your emotions are saying. When you feel complete, move on to the next direction.

Honor your body. What do you need physically? What is your body feeling, asking for, or wanting? How is your energy level? Are you rested? What type of movement do you need? How can you move your body today so it feels nurtured? What is it craving nutritionally?

Listen to what you need to hear, opening up to the wisdom of your body.

Now take out your journal and write down what you just discovered.

Close your ritual by expressing your gratitude. Then, commit to honoring one of your needs.

Now that we've laid a solid foundation, we'll begin to decode the natal chart and how its core elements—your moon sign, sun sign, and rising sign—affect your cosmic health.

Part III

AIR

Integrating Your Core Astrology

Creation Myths the world over begin with chaos, but the original meaning of the word "chaos" did not imply confusion and turmoil. Rather it simply meant the infinite void.

—Demetra George, from *Mysteries of the Dark Moon*

CHAPTER 5

The Moon Sign

Learning How to Self-Nurture

We tend to glorify being the "first" in our family—the first to attend college, the first to leave that small town   but being a first wasn't easy for my mom. Feeling unfulfilled as a stay-at-home mother of three in the 1980s, when more women were working outside the home, she yearned to have her own career. My mom soon became the first woman in my family to start her own business *and* the first to get divorced. Unfortunately, this amplified a deep-seated, decades-long rift with her own mother.

In many ways the iconic Italian grandmother, mine was a devoted homemaker who had emigrated from Italy at age six and never had her own driver's license. While she lived in the same state as my mother, they were seemingly worlds apart. My mom's insistence on pursuing her independence made no sense to my grandmother, especially when my mom's decision to work led to a contentious divorce from my dad.

It was a heavy burden to carry in my patriarchal Italian family. That pattern of what I call "double rejection"—my grandmother feeling rejected by my mom's decisions, and my mom then feeling rejected by my grandmother—is one that eventually trickled down into my own relationship with my mom.

After my hysterectomy, my mom desperately wanted me to follow my doctors' advice. "Just do what they tell you to," she'd plead with me. Looking back, her insistence that the doctors knew best was understandable, but I was determined to heal my own way. Instead of doing what she (and the doctors) asked, I flew thousands of miles away, literally to the opposite coast, to find healing—not to mention myself—on my own terms.

For years that decision created so much tension between us that we could barely communicate. It was deeply painful—and ultimately *the* emotional fault line that led me toward the most important healing work I've ever done: my work with the moon.

The moon also connects us to our maternal instincts as well as our matrilineal heritage, both of which can have significant healing effects on our relationships and our lives.

In this chapter, we'll look at your natal moon sign and how it can help you nourish yourself emotionally as well as physically and spiritually. First, let's look at some of the science and astrology around our emotions and how we're connected to the people who came before us.

Accessing Your Emotional Landscape

Your emotional health influences and shifts in tandem with your physical health—remember, *everything is connected.*

Beyond the mind–body connection, emotional wellness guides key behaviors and decision-making that can have lasting physical, social, and professional consequences. How we engage with indulgence, restriction, creativity, impulsivity, generosity, intimacy, and genius—to name just a few—have an equally profound impact on our health and our lives.

At the core of our emotional, mental, and therefore physical well-being are the thousands of thoughts and emotions we experience each day. For true emotional health, we need to be able to handle and express all emotions in a healthy way. This means that positive emotions, like joy and excitement, *as well as* negative emotions, like anxiety and fear, all need to be expressed. While positive emotions may sound more inviting, as Brené Brown has famously asserted, joy is often the emotion we're most afraid to feel, as it can seem to foreshadow disappointment, rejection, even crisis.[1]

Given that even positive emotions aren't easy to feel and process—plus the fact that we continuously cycle through a vast, often overwhelming range of emotions—it's no wonder our relationship with our emotions is fraught. Combined with how much we do each day, how many people are in our lives, the many responsibilities and interactions we have, there's a lot of emotion to manage in any given hour, day, or week!

Not surprisingly, most of us are prone to experiencing internal tension from feeling so much emotion that we're unable and unwilling to express. To mask the roller-coaster ride our emotions can take us on, we resort to using superficial language. When asked how we are, we reply that we're "good" or "fine." Most of the time, we deliver these words reflexively, giving little conscious thought to what we're saying. Then, eager to avoid having to say more, we quickly add, "How are you?"

However rote, even meaningless, these exchanges may be at times, it's also true that most neighbors, coworkers, and even friends don't typically have the time or deep interest needed to listen to the nuances of our lives, like our worries about an upcoming job interview or our excitement about a new relationship.

But also, how often do we say "good" or "fine" in part because we don't know how we're actually feeling? Let's be honest: we don't often have the time or bandwidth to pay attention to our own feelings, let alone understand them. We instead go through life from a more intellectual place, strategizing what needs to get done next, thinking about the future or the past, itemizing to-dos instead of sensing or emoting.

On top of all of this, the noise of other people's emotions can crowd out our own. There are also times when we simply choose not to recognize what we're feeling because it's too overwhelming or painful. We ignore those emotions or tuck them deep, deep down because it allows us to get on with our day.

Nothing Left to Fear Except Fear Itself

I'll say it once again, both because it's that critical and because we so often forget it: emotions are *impermanent*. Even if they arrive with a vengeance, when we present ourselves to them, understand what they are asking us to acknowledge, and find healthy ways to express them, they transform, making room for other emotions. Instead of avoiding and suppressing emotion, it's far better to notice and honor our emotional ebbs and flows. The sooner we admit what we're really feeling, the quicker we can transform less desirable emotional states into more appealing and productive ones.

Emotions are neither good nor bad. For example, feeling envy toward a friend or a loved one occasionally is a natural emotion. It's part of human nature; there's nothing inherently good or bad about it. The same is true when it comes to experiencing anger, depression, or anxiety. In the words of my positive psychology teacher, Dr. Tal Ben-Shahar, "The question is how do I choose to behave, to act, as a result of it [a strong emotion]? That's where the moral domain enters. That's where I can have moral or immoral behavior."[2] Feeling all of our emotions, even the difficult ones, like anger, hatred, and jealously, is essential to our health, well-being, and happiness. It's our actions and reactions that have ramifications, not our emotions alone.

Trusting the impermanence and wisdom of emotions also allows us to find comfort in constant change. It helps us let go of the urge to stifle, amplify, or control. Instead, we can let our emotions appear and express exactly as they are—and we can then grow stronger and more resilient in the process of feeling and releasing them.

Our emotions remain our most intimate landscape. They have a language all their own, and the only way we learn it is by listening to them.

LOCATING EMOTIONS IN YOUR BODY

I often lead my clients through this exercise to access their emotions:

Close your eyes and scan your body, noticing what sensations you feel in your body. Whether out loud or silently in your mind, focus on one sensation and describe it. Now give it a color and a name. Take a few deep breaths and ask the sensation if it has a message for you.

By placing so much attention on one sensation, and then communicating with whatever emotion(s) may be behind it, you can better understand what it is asking you to express. From there you can see how to constructively process the feeling coming up. Instead of lashing out in anger, for instance, you might explain to a trusted loved one that he or she hurt your feelings. Alternatively, you could use mindfulness or journaling to down-regulate stress. Developing emotional literacy inevitably enhances your well-being and boosts your resilience.

Your Moon Sign and Your Emotional Needs

As important as it is to access your many emotions, practicing emotional awareness amidst the chaos of daily life can be overwhelming. What I love about moon work—attuning to your natal moon sign and the ongoing lunar cycle—is how it allows you to navigate this otherwise challenging undertaking with more ease and self-compassion.

Your natal moon sign reflects the emotional core of your being: your deeper needs and what you require to feel emotionally satisfied and secure. Developing an understanding of your moon sign helps you to cultivate emotional self-awareness. As just one brief example, having your natal moon in Virgo means that your deepest need is to feel that you are being of service. However, to feed this drive and make an impact in people's lives, you also need ample alone time to recover.

Once you're aware of your emotional needs, you can determine if you're living in alignment with them, and then make any adjustments necessary to meet those needs. That will boost your emotional well-being and, in turn, your physical health.

Connecting to your lunar needs will also link you to a strategy for your health that aligns with your actual needs rather than the needs you think you should have or the needs of others.

YOUR GRANDMOTHER LIVES ON... INSIDE YOU?

The science of epigenetics, which illuminates how DNA is expressed, reveals that our choices — what we eat and drink, how much we exercise, the levels of stress we're under, as well as the trauma we've experienced, including the trauma we inherited from our ancestry through our genetics, and much more — affect our children's, and even our grandchildren's, health and well-being.

Along similar lines, some findings suggest that ovaries develop in utero. This means that those of us who were assigned the gender female at birth may be more closely genetically related to our grandmothers than science previously understood.

Combined, these findings underscore the transgenerational impact of health, especially around how we care for our health and mental/emotional well-being.

This process also works in reverse, of course, and on the psyche as well as the body. As a result, your mother's relationship to her body, and all of her life experiences, likely affects how you relate to your own. Additionally, the way you were (or weren't) nurtured by your mother often influences how you nurture (or fail to nurture) yourself.

This science also underscores the importance of healing racialized trauma, which is genetically passed on and perpetuated from generation to generation. To learn more, I highly suggest checking out the book by Resmaa Menakem *My Grandmother's Hands: Racialized Trauma and the Pathway to Mending Our Hearts and Bodies*. In it he writes the following: "We tend to think of healing as something binary: either we are broken or we are healed from that brokenness. But that's not how healing operates, and it's almost never how human growth works. More often, healing and growth take place on a continuum, with innumerable points between utter brokenness and total health."[3]

Take a moment and consider this: what stories, ways of being, fears, and pain are you carrying that you inherited from your blood line? The answer may elude you right now. Be patient. But know this: as you heal yourself, you may vacillate between brokenness and health, but by cultivating your resilience and not giving up, you are healing your grandmother too. Remember, everything is connected!

The Moon: One of Your Closest Confidantes

In astrology, your moon sign is the zodiac sign occupied by the moon at the moment of your birth. The moon visits each sign approximately every two-and-a-half days on its near-monthly cycle of waxing and waning. This is why an Aquarius born on January 22 may be very different from an Aquarius born on January 25.

The moon has long been associated with transformation and the feminine, and the moon's phases of new, full, and "old" were thought by ancient cultures to represent the phases of a woman's life as maiden, mother, and crone. And of course, as discussed in chapter 3, the moon's approximately twenty-nine-and-a-half-day cycle from new moon to new moon closely matches the menstrual cycle. The moon directs the ebb and flow of the tides and mirrors the timing of menstruation, and it's not surprising that the moon is so closely tied to fluctuating emotions too.

Our connection to the moon runs just as deep, and is just as powerful, as our dance with the sun. Think of the moon as expressing your private inner world, while the sun expresses who you are—your identity and vitality. The moon is your yin, your more tenderhearted qualities, such as nurturance, sensitivity, and caring. The sun is your yang, your daytime energy, representing traits of assertiveness and independence. Out mostly at night, the moon reflects your nighttime energy, a quiet, private time of sleeping, dreaming, and nourishing your body and mind.

Using Desire to Create Momentum

Knowing what you need is knowing what you want, and there's no more powerful emotion than desire. If you're an Aries sun or moon who needs lots of exercise to feel emotionally strong and secure, you're going to want to make time to go to that spin class, take that hiking trip, and learn how to rock climb. That may mean carving out time in your schedule and saying no to obligations that would prevent you from working out. It means prioritizing your emotional needs and honoring your desires.

The beauty of knowing what you want, which in this case is ample time for physical expression, is that you also discover what you don't want and what's least likely to satisfy you. While writing a book may nourish a Gemini, who is here to teach, an Aries, on the other hand, may lack patience for such a long-winded, time-consuming project. The aim is to recognize that as part of your emotional makeup.

So often we walk through life thinking that what works for others should work for us too. *Stability makes her happy. It should make me happy too.* But when you try to be steadier, more consistent—sticking it out in a job or a relationship—you don't feel happy, you feel frustrated. You may go on like that, trying out what seems to make other people happy instead of acknowledging your emotional needs. In this example, stability may not be it for you; adventure and novelty may be what lights your emotional and spiritual fire.

By honoring your desires, you can see if you're in a situation that's good for you, and then care for yourself in a way that supports happiness. It will help you to uncover exactly what you need to feel emotionally nourished and then take action to make it happen.

Making It Happen: My Prayers Answered

In 2006, five years after I began living in alignment with the phases of the moon, I sold everything I owned, sublet my 350-square-foot studio in San Francisco, and boarded a one-way flight to Europe. While I'd spent two years preparing for this adventure, I intentionally had no real itinerary and minimal specific travel plans. My goal was bold — to circumnavigate the globe without using a single credit card, utilizing nothing more than the intensity of my desire and my intuition as my way forward. It would be the ultimate backpacking adventure. On this trip, I planned to employ everything I had learned about being the magician of my own life to see how it would turn out.

With the exception of a couple of close friends, no one in my life thought the trip was a good idea. From several standpoints — finances, health, and safety, for starters — the trip was a daring move, to say the least. Yet to me it felt healing. Many luminaries had taught me that repressed emotion can contribute to disease in the body. I believed that was the case for me, and by honoring a critical emotion — desire — I was able to use it to shape-shift a new reality. I practiced this like my life depended on it. Because, frankly, it did.

Making a firm decision to take that trip also allowed me to unlock massive momentum in my life. For reasons that defied logic, doors previously closed to me began to open. In preparation for my trip, I was able to pay down debt and save almost five thousand dollars, which was a huge feat at that point. Also, just before my first flight out of New York, I got bumped off my flight. The airline gave me a hotel room, meal vouchers, and a $400 travel gift certificate. Jackpot! My backpacker's travel budget had just gotten a very welcome helping hand. It was one of the many times when I would be blessed with cosmic sweetness.

Honoring My Desires

While my world tour encompassed many profoundly magical moments, one in particular still stands out. I was in my third month of traveling, and it was mid-July. Standing in front of the Prado National Museum in Madrid, Spain, dripping sweat while wearing a heavy backpack, I began overthinking where to sleep. As I indulged in a fit of excessive rumination, I suddenly had an epiphany. I realized that I literally couldn't make a wrong decision so long as I followed my intuition and stayed true to my desire. (Duh.) In that moment, I tapped into an emotion I'd so rarely felt but desperately wanted... *freedom.*

In that hot, ridiculously obsessive moment, I genuinely got it: no matter what I chose, if I didn't like it, I could change it again. Feeling that newfound freedom and permission to act on my *intuition* ended a limiting pattern of control and fear that had haunted me for years.

From that point onward, I committed to relaxing even more into the experiment at hand: traveling alone internationally for months with zero plans. By allowing myself to manage discomfort, I freed myself to take risks and trust my intuition. In the course of my travels, I also learned how to self-soothe, self-nurture, and bounce back from disappointment.

With each new experience and each new day, I deepened my connection to myself and my emotional needs. The serendipity was so ever-present on that trip, I gained an abiding trust in it and my inner guidance. Ever since, my intuition has played an even bigger starring role in my identity and my life.

Deciding to go on that trip was monumental, but even more so was the decision to take a radical level of responsibility for my own healing, not just physically but emotionally. Whether I liked it or not, being emotionally well meant living my life on my terms, not just when that came easily but also when it meant taking huge risks that weren't guaranteed to work out the way I desired.

The Power of Choice and Desire

The power to decide is by far the most significant power you have. All choices, and especially bold choices, generate synchronicity. Even when a decision seems "wrong," as I realized that day in Madrid, you always have the option to make a new and different decision. Regardless, the process of deciding, of choosing, fuels your growth and development like little else can. Just by making a choice and chasing down your desires, you will get better at nurturing yourself.

Choose something real, something radical, something that heals you on an emotional level. Then commit to making it happen—no matter what. That's how you, how any of us, realize your most fulfilling and inspiring life. Almost without exception, that process begins with emotion. It starts with getting in touch with your deeper desires. Your emotions are raw power. They fuel you and allow you to conjure the reality you most desire to live.

Your natal moon sign will help you decode the language of your emotions and build your resilience, both of which are essential to taking the risks required to step into a bigger version of yourself. As you become more comfortable with honoring your desires, you'll develop self-esteem based on an appreciation for your inherent value, not one based on what other people think of you or how they evaluate you.

The Moon in Your Natal Chart: Putting It to Work for You

Aside from the moon's transits (which I walked you through in chapter 3), understanding your natal moon—where the moon was at the time of your birth, also known as your moon sign—helps you to understand your emotional disposition. It illuminates what you need to feel emotionally satiated.

Physically, the moon is also connected to the stomach. Learning to work with the moon can help you "stomach" your emotions and understand how they affect your body, and vice versa. This also helps you to unlock distress tolerance, which is the ability to sit with difficult emotions.

Remember, the moon represents your subconscious and emotional needs.

Tuning in to your own personal moon sign is essential to understanding and accessing the raw power of your feelings, your emotional essence.

DON'T HAVE YOUR NATAL CHART?

Throughout the rest of this book, you'll want a copy of your natal chart to put each planet's purpose and directive into a more personal context. To get the most accurate version of your chart, you'll need your birth date, time of birth, and place of birth. If you don't have your time of birth, you can get a natal chart that either excludes your rising sign (discussed in chapter 7) or estimates it. To learn how to get a free copy of your chart, visit JenniferRacioppi.com /resources.

The following are lists of qualities of each moon sign.

NATAL MOON IN ARIES ♈

Pioneer. Director. Athlete.

Symbol: Ram
Element: Fire
Ruling Planet: Mars
Mode: Cardinal

If you're born with the moon in Aries, you have a Mars-ruled moon, which means that you're an initiator who feels most energized when getting things started. Action-oriented by nature, you have an incredible presence. However, you're learning about patience and follow-through. With your natal moon in super-independent Aries, you have no interest in abiding by authority figures who haven't earned their keep (unless you're the one calling the shots). Small talk and niceties don't do it for you either.

Your Aries moon is more of a warrior than a worrier, but you can be afraid of finding yourself trapped by outside circumstances. You tend to act on your impulse to keep pushing forward. People can always rely on you to cut to the chase. Just be careful you aren't cutting to the quick too.

With so much fire, be mindful of your impatience, which can generate excessive anger. Finding outlets for your bold energy is key — mindfulness practices, like meditation, as well as heart-pumping cardio, can help you in this area.

While you like to take matters into your own hands and your tolerance for hardship is as tough as nails, remember, you were never meant to be a one-person show. Learning to delegate is one of the most important things you can do for your emotional health!

Aries rules the head. Cultivate patience and manage stress wisely so you can bring your goals to fruition without any headaches.

NATAL MOON IN TAURUS ♉

Epicurean. Gardener. Aphrodite.

Symbol: Bull
Element: Earth
Ruling Planet: Venus
Mode: Fixed

The moon is exalted in Taurus, which means it functions with excellence in this sign. With a natal moon in Taurus, you naturally cultivate a sense of peacefulness and serenity.

For you, nourishing and nurturing come as easily as breathing. You innately understand what someone needs, and you're more than willing to give it to them, whether that means whipping up comfort cookies or connecting during a tea for two. Don't be surprised if you find that the people around you tend to seek out your support. With your Taurus moon, you can't help but exude the vibe of grounded stability.

When it comes to comfort, the Taurus moon sign rules the physical plane — what you can taste, touch, and smell — which for you is a way of understanding the world and your own soul. You easily see the natural interplay between the rhythms of nature and your own body, and you know how to put them to use.

While you're happiest when dealing with the physical realm, you're more than a softhearted — and let's be real, fairly stubborn — soul. Make a point of dipping into the inner emotional waters of your opposite sign, Scorpio. You may be surprised how deep your internal resources go.

Taurus rules the throat, so speak your truth. You may even want to sing to keep your throat clear.

NATAL MOON IN GEMINI ♊

Networker. Teacher. Writer.

Symbol: Twins
Element: Air
Ruling Planet: Mercury
Mode: Mutable

With a natal moon in Gemini, you are wired to communicate. You don't quite feel like yourself unless you're gathering data from people around you and then sharing what you've learned with others. Since you're a natural teacher, self-expression feeds your soul's urge to communicate important information and gives your eclectic mind a sense of purpose.

Yet your social nature can contribute to burnout. Know your red flags, which include mood swings, anxiety, and acute depression. The key to your emotional health lies in your deep need to *disconnect*.

Screen-free alone time may initially feel unnatural, even isolating, but with sufficient practice, you'll discover that it's more valuable than gold in terms of your emotional well-being.

With so many ideas and so much information running through your agile mind, you may quickly move from one project to the next. Ultimately, it's your sense of purpose that will prevent you from spreading yourself too thin and bouncing from one priority to the next without completing either. You've got the ability to gain a rare glimpse at ideas ready to be made manifest. Choose the ones that light you up and see them all the way through.

Gemini corresponds with the arms, hands, and shoulders, so seek out physical practices that help you get calm and remain focused. Think transformational breath work, hatha yoga, or strength training.

NATAL MOON IN CANCER ♋

Empress. Breadwinner. Nurturer.

Symbol: Crab
Element: Water
Ruling Planet: Moon
Mode: Cardinal

With a natal moon in Cancer, your emotional intuition has a depth that's truly beyond logical knowing. You feel everything to the max, but are you using that emotional impact to evolve more deeply into yourself?

While you feel fulfilled when caring for others, caring for yourself is an equally important way to build the security your soul craves. No matter how much you nurture, you can't control what happens to the people and things you love, but you'll always be with yourself. For you it's #selfcareorbust.

The key is to know when it's time to slow down and recharge or get moving and charge forward. When it's the former, give yourself the time and space to putter around the house or use solo time to reboot in another way. Just make sure to get back out into the world when you're ready to face your dreams head-on. In fact, take a cue from your opposite sign, Capricorn, and don't be afraid to take up space!

Your emotional health relies on your ability to develop your sense of personal security. This means that confidence, self-assurance, and financial security are critical. Don't underestimate the power of healing family dynamics either. Looking at issues in your family through a historical lens and working through them in therapy might add potency to your healing.

As the moon changes signs, pay attention to how you feel. A Cancer moon can be a bit moody, so learning to understand and predict your emotional fluctuations gives you an advantage!

Cancer correlates with the chest and breast. Keeping a journal where you can get things "off your chest" will help you to process your emotions in a healthy way.

NATAL MOON IN LEO ♌

Sovereign. Motivator. Leader.

Symbol: Lion
Element: Fire
Ruling Planet: Sun
Mode: Fixed

With Leo as your moon sign, you aren't short on warmth and affection. As a lion-hearted soul, you are meant to embody and embrace a brave and bold heart. That courage, more than anything, will empower you to take a stand.

While you have a deep need to be seen, you're not necessarily motivated by the spotlight for its own sake. Though let's be honest: you often find yourself in the spotlight anyway. You feel your best when you can project your generous spirit into your environment and the hearts of those you love.

Sheer fun is key to your well-being and health, as are emotional and creative self-expression. There's nothing you love more than showing those you love where you've been or what fresh and colorful thing you've created. While sharing can be nourishing, it's important to build emotional resilience around what brings your lion heart joy—even when, and especially when, no one is watching. Go ahead, make fun and fulfilling art. Write those songs and screenplays. Share those epic ideas. But remember to give yourself the space and time to channel your light into creative pursuits that fill you up even *before* you share them with others.

Alone time will do your emotional health wonders. With Leo ruling the heart and upper back, it's essential to stand tall and pay attention to your posture.

NATAL MOON IN VIRGO ♍

Mentor. Engineer. Editor.

Symbol: Virgin
Element: Earth
Ruling Planet: Mercury
Mode: Mutable

When your moon sign falls in Virgo, you tend to gain emotional stability from your routine and your physical surroundings. You are here to serve others. So as long as you have purpose in your work, you are good to go. You don't need luxe decor or lavender oil brewing in the diffuser. You need the simplicity that allows you to focus on what you love most. The more you have everything in its proper place, the more at peace you feel.

While you thrive in situations where everything lines up the way you think it should, this tendency to sort, shuffle, and repeat can get in the way of tapping into your true emotions. You're pretty sensitive when it comes down to it, and you hold a lot of your anxieties in your stomach. Cry, laugh, scream—do what's both necessary and therapeutic to let it all go every once in a while. Free yourself from rigid expectations and channel the strengths of your opposite sign, Pisces, for an intuitive download. Now *that's* streamlining.

And while you're loosening up a bit, make sure you turn that urge to serve toward yourself also. Give your own big-picture desires as much time and attention as you do your itemized to-do lists and watch as the magic unfolds.

Since Virgo rules your abdomen and much of the digestive process, stay mindful of your diet. Gut-healing protocols will help you feel balanced and on point.

NATAL MOON IN LIBRA ♎

Artist. Advocate. Liberator.

Symbol: Scales
Element: Air
Ruling Planet: Venus
Mode: Cardinal

As a Libra moon, you feel best when your life is balanced. From your friendships to your career, you prefer for everyone to chill and everything to be chill.

But that's not how life works. You need to learn to navigate the unpleasant emotions that make us all human in order to find your equilibrium from within the storm. Accepting less harmonious emotions in the moment is the key to developing long-term resilience. Let yourself go deeper sometimes — to feel it *all*. Then, do what you do best, and find the beauty in it.

Remember, too, that more than any other moon sign, the dictum "Know who you are and be who you are" applies to you. Libra is both an air sign and a cardinal one. While balance is an innate priority, there's nothing docile about you. Learning to fight for what you believe in is essential. You are driven by a sense of justice and here to make the world a more equitable place for all.

It may seem paradoxical to find yourself through others, but by interacting with, learning from, and loving others, you figure out how to help people liberate themselves. That said, self-expression through art, fashion, and design gives you a platform to animate your sophisticated knowing.

Libra rules the lumbar region. To stay healthy, build your core strength, and resist the urge to constantly twist yourself into a pretzel for others. Your lumbar spine will thank you!

NATAL MOON IN SCORPIO ♏

Sorceress. Therapist. Investigator.

Symbol: Scorpion
Element: Water
Ruling Planets: Pluto and Mars
Mode: Fixed

As a Scorpio moon, "intensity" is your middle name. Yet you aren't into drama for drama's sake. In fact, that will deflate you faster than a pinhole in a balloon. Instead, your intensity derives from your search for truth.

You're at your best when you go deep. Having a wide circle of friends feels pointless if your time together is devoid of soul-stirring conversation. Intimacy, both with yourself and others, is essential.

Allow yourself to honor your intuition and explore your own nature, but remember that we weren't all blessed with your ability to "see through the veil." You ask a lot from loved ones. Be mindful that not everyone possesses the ability to see themselves as you do. Honor where people are, and accept them as is rather than pushing them into your depths.

You aren't into sugarcoating, mostly because you already know that playing nice doesn't serve anyone. You'd rather not waste time when you could dive deeper and discover what makes someone tick. Unlike other signs, you don't fear what you'll uncover. You figure that even if you stumble upon something unbearable, at least you'll know the truth before it can damage your sensitive soul.

Scorpio rules the pelvic region, which houses the reproductive system and the rectum. Therefore, it's helpful to pay close attention to reproductive health as well as to make sure you're eliminating regularly. (Yes, I am talking about poop!) Unlocking your erotic power is extremely important for you too.

NATAL MOON IN SAGITTARIUS ♐

Bon Vivant. Teacher. Truth Seeker.

Symbol: Archer
Element: Fire
Ruling Planet: Jupiter
Mode: Mutable

There are few people who are as fun to be around as those with a Sagittarius moon. Like all fire signs, you're passionate about what you love, but for you in particular, that translates into unwavering optimism and a general sense of well-being.

To stay in emotional alignment, you need to connect your sense of goodwill with your highest truth. How can you serve others with your vision and creativity? How can you be true to your own ethical standards *and* express your joy? These are the kinds of questions that will keep your emotions buoyed, even when things get hard.

By giving yourself permission to express your truth, you free yourself from anything that isn't in alignment with who you really are. And when you break free, you give others permission to do the same.

Throughout the inevitable highs and lows of life, it's important that you stay open, honest, and connected to your emotions.

While all fire signs need regular stimulation to feed their soul, you need it most of all. Since you're prone to restlessness when you feel bored or stagnant, make a point of seeking out adventure, even if that means you're just taking a different route to work on occasion.

Sagittarius rules the hips and thighs, so yoga asanas are great because they help you to feel your emotions. Think pigeon pose, and psoas muscle stretches.

NATAL MOON IN CAPRICORN ♑

Expert. Strategist. Executive.

Symbol: Sea Goat
Element: Earth
Ruling Planet: Saturn
Mode: Cardinal

With a natal moon in Capricorn, you're not one to wear your heart on your sleeve. In fact, you may sometimes wonder why everyone gets torn up over everything from rom-coms to the state of the world.

It's not that you don't care; it's just not in your nature to dwell on a problem. You're most emotionally satisfied when you're *doing* something to create a kinder, more thoughtful world—bonus points if it involves resolving complex issues.

While you appreciate reaching the top, it's important to pay equal attention to how you feel when you're in the middle of the climb. Of all the moon signs, you're most likely to stuff down your feelings and endure straight-up BS in the name of goals. You'll deal with it when you get there, you tell yourself. Yet with your drive and work ethic, you'll always be striving for the next level. To feel emotionally nourished, you need to learn to play, wander, and explore during, not after, that long climb to the tippy top.

Ruled by authoritarian Saturn, you don't take responsibilities lightly. You're here to learn what it means to fulfill your responsibilities, even when—especially when—the process requires inordinate amounts of patience and perseverance.

Capricorn rules knees, so pay extra attention to the structures and foundations of your life. Strength training and alignment-based workouts encourage your power and determination.

NATAL MOON IN AQUARIUS ♒

Genius. Revolutionary. Designer.

Symbol: Water Bearer
Element: Air
Ruling Planets: Saturn and Uranus
Mode: Fixed

With your natal moon in the sign of the water bearer, you spend way more time *thinking* about your emotions than experiencing them. Your internal satisfaction comes more from generating and connecting ideas. You derive joy from big-picture, long-term projects, especially if you can bring in diverse thinkers to help foster a new perspective.

As an air sign with your modern ruler being revolutionary Uranus, you're a thought leader with an impeccable ability to puzzle your way through problems. While your unique perspective is a much-needed gift, it can be hard for you to relate to others at times. When you feel restricted or disrespected, you may isolate yourself instead of inviting people into your point of view.

You tend to see humanity as a collective instead of taking a closer look at each person as an individual. While this can make you seem aloof, it's also an opportunity to develop more intimacy with others, as well as yourself. You are here for liberation—your liberation and the liberation of all beings *everywhere*. This requires embracing intimacy.

To feel satisfied on this strange and sometimes cumbersome planet, it's key for you to fully accept what makes you, *you*. Your innovative, progressive ideas lend themselves to wild flashes of insight that may ping in your chest when you're on the right track. Write them down—*all* of them—and give them space to marinate.

Aquarius rules the ankles, so do your best to stay balanced. Practice balancing via a skateboard, snowboard, or paddleboard, or even try a pogo stick!

NATAL MOON IN PISCES ♓

Empath. Healer. Poet.

Symbol: Pair of Fish
Element: Water
Ruling Planets: Neptune and Jupiter
Mode: Mutable

With a natal Pisces moon, you're born a wise old soul. Even from a young age, you possess wisdom it might take the rest of us a lifetime (or several) to uncover.

As a mutable water sign, sensing the surrounding energy fields of people and places is as easy as breathing. As powerful as this ability is, it can also make you prone to emotional ebbs and flows. You may sometimes struggle to differentiate between your emotional energy and that of the people around you.

Being so intuitively "plugged in," you aren't satisfied with a "normal" life. By regularly transcending your physical body and touching down on the energy fields of others, you can escape your own limitations and experience a wider, multidimensional world. This is like a balm for your overstimulated soul.

You possess the sage-like wisdom needed to change hearts and minds. Between your creative intuition and the depths of your empathy, you have tremendous gifts to share with the world. Give yourself permission to drop the dogmatic baggage and rise.

Pay keen attention to your intuition and feelings. While your emotional intelligence is off the charts, beware of codependency. Learning boundaries is key!

Pisces rules the feet, so regular foot massages, or even foot reflexology, are important ways of grounding your ethereal energy. This helps you hold your boundaries with others, by feeling grounded in yourself.

The Moon and Mothering

Given how deeply connected the moon sign is to our nurturing, of both ourselves and others, I want to share another story about mothering. Unlike my own story, which focuses on matrilineal heritage, this client's story is about herself as a mother to her very young son.

Still breastfeeding her child when she came to me, Carina worried that her diet might be causing her baby's painful skin condition. Committed to using only natural medicine, she'd sought out several practitioners to help her find a solution. One doctor put her on an extremely restrictive eating plan. Already a vegetarian for religious reasons (she is an Indian woman who practices Jainism), she felt frustrated and increasingly angry that, in addition to birthing and breastfeeding her baby, she now couldn't eat most of the foods she enjoyed. Feeling irritated by the constraints being placed on her, she soon began fighting with her husband, seething with resentment that so much of the caretaking was falling on her.

As I listened to Carina's story and helped her to understand her natal chart, she began to see that this restrictive diet wasn't going to work. With her natal moon in Leo, she couldn't sacrifice all of her needs. Being deprived of pleasure runs counter to her emotional well-being. Not being able to eat the foods she enjoyed wouldn't work for her. As a mother doing so much of the nurturing her newborn demanded, her Leo moon awoke within her the need to establish a boundary and voice her needs!

That realization prompted her to have her son tested for allergies. Since learning that he is allergic to a few specific foods, she's been able to alter her diet to exclude just those foods, which has in turn allowed her to eat all others. As a result, she's been able to restore her emotional equilibrium. That has had a hugely positive impact on her marriage.

Our emotions are in many ways the foundation of our health, and by honoring them, we become more astute in our pursuit of solutions.

THE LUNAR NODES

Metaphorically, I think of the nodes as intersections along two highways in the sky. The highway of the moon's path around the earth crosses the highway of the apparent path (celestial equator) of the sun around the earth.
— DIETRECH J. PESSIN, FROM *LUNAR SHADOWS III*

The lunar nodes are where the plane of the moon's orbit intersects with the plane of the ecliptic. They are not planets or celestial bodies, nor are they observable in the sky. No less, they play an important role in your chart.

The *north node* ☊ represents the challenges to conquer to develop into your fullest self. While intimidating at first, the themes of the north node reveal where you can find immense fulfillment and satisfaction, if only you put yourself on, and adhere to, the path of growth. The north node represents character traits you are developing and the fate you are claiming.

The *south node* ☋, conversely, signals where you've been: the lessons and strengths that you naturally possess or, if you subscribe to the theory of reincarnation, what you bring with you from a past life. Your south node themes reveal how you tend to approach life: the innate, comfort-zone qualities that (from some perspectives) you may fall back on as a safety blanket and that, when unchallenged, may hold you back.

Together, the north node and the south node indicate a polarity, as they are always found directly opposite each other on the natal chart, in opposing signs. This nodal axis reminds us of the ever-present duality that shows up in our lives. We can see each node as simultaneously contradictory and complementary, incomplete without the other. The north node is where you are assimilating new opportunities and creativity. In contrast, the south node indicates where you need to discharge undesirable ways of being and liberate yourself from habitual ways of being that no longer serve you.[4] The goal remains to move toward the attributes you are developing (north node), and when you find yourself relying on qualities that feel safe and secure, or you are caught in a rut (south node), to choose the path of growth over the familiar.

From a practical standpoint, this underscores the importance of moving beyond the comforts of your south node and using those strengths as a jumping-off point for success indicated by your north node potential.

One of my favorite books available on this topic is by Jan Spiller. *Astrology for the Soul* serves as an in-depth exploration of the nodes. Also, Meira Epstein, a faculty member of the New York National Council for Geocosmic Research, offers a riveting perspective on this topic. If you ever get the chance to study with her or hear her speak, do!

The Nodes in Transit

You can also look to the nodal axis of the present day to see which areas of duality the universe is asking us to address. For instance, at the time of the release of this book, the nodes of fate will be on the Gemini-Sagittarius axis, which asks us to harmonize our ideology and philosophy: how we communicate, conceptualize community, and share ideas (north node in Gemini), as well as pursue the healing of historically held-back liberation (south node in Sagittarius). The moon's nodes are important, as they indicate the signs where eclipses will happen.

The Nodes in Your Natal Chart

Here are *very* brief explanations of what your nodal axis might indicate in your life. Take this as a jumping-off point!

North Node in Aries, South Node in Libra: You are asked to rise to your Aries-inspired independence and leadership, which means learning to be assertive and confident, trusting fully in yourself. While you may lean on your relationships for guidance and decision-making, cultivate your sovereignty and independence. Stay mindful of codependent dynamics.

North Node in Libra, South Node in Aries: You are here to develop partnerships and make waves in the direction of peace. Use art, fashion, beauty, and devout commitment to justice to enrich your life. To offset a proclivity toward impatience and impulsivity, meditate. There is an immense opportunity for growth when you partner up, ask for feedback, and consider the ideas and needs of others.

North Node in Taurus, South Node in Scorpio: Look to develop your intrinsic self-worth and enjoy moments of peace. Nurture yourself mindfully with food and pleasure. Spending time in nature elevates you. You may notice a tendency to attract intensity and crisis, and be consumed by the needs and troubles of others as a source of self-worth. You are learning trust.

North Node in Scorpio, South Node in Taurus: Lean into the natural changes in life; these are the moments that bring the deep vulnerability, intimacy, and transformation that will ultimately put you on a more authentic course. Be careful not to hold too tightly to the possessions, people, and ideas that bring you security. Own your sexual prowess. There's nothing wrong with being a bit intense.

North Node in Gemini, South Node in Sagittarius: As a natural teacher, you are here to spread knowledge and wisdom. Your strong opinions and viewpoints allow you to lead with exceptional power, yet stay mindful of a tendency to be a bit abrupt. Ground your conviction by slowing down, listening with grace, and seeking the open exchange of ideas with others. Listen to hear, not to respond.

North Node in Sagittarius, South Node in Gemini: With an adept communication capacity, you are a master at expressing yourself. Yet you tend to become mentally overstimulated and sometimes so overextended that you override your intuition with logic and lose sight of the bigger picture. Build your faith in your intuition and follow your inclinations to seek adventure and physical fitness. Stay mindful of gossip and devoted to the truth.

North Node in Cancer, South Node in Capricorn: You are here to master the art of giving and receiving nourishment. Yet your natural ambition may cause you to feel like you always need to be in control. As you achieve a more profound sense of your spirituality and a real sense of safety and security, look at where you can loosen the reins and show your vulnerability. Prioritize your personal life and family.

North Node in Capricorn, South Node in Cancer: You find inspiration and leadership and expand creatively when you take responsibility for your life. Look at where you can accept more responsibility and take ownership of your life. That's where you'll find the robust security you desire. You have an innate capacity for nourishing and nurturing others and are developing a stalwart, brass-tacks approach to business and life. For you, genius is the right use of a work ethic.

North Node in Leo, South Node in Aquarius: You may love standing out from the crowd, especially if it means you get to go for what you want. As you learn to prioritize yourself, you give others the freedom to do the same. "Freedom" is a key word for you. The challenge? Sometimes your rebellious nature means you give up or check out too soon. Learning to stick with your dreams is what you need to become the most resilient version of yourself.

North Node in Aquarius, South Node in Leo: Break away from the pack and follow your authentic path. Resist the need for approval and instead take risks on behalf of what you know to be true. Stay dogged when it comes to honoring your values and working on behalf of social change. You are here to encourage freedom. Yet you need to be wary of your own ego. You can easily get looped into the "disease to please," especially when you accept another person's love as the basis of your self-respect.

North Node in Virgo, South Node in Pisces: With your south node in Pisces, you have a deep faith that the universe will provide, which may lead you to "wing it" without a plan. Learn to co-create with the universe by meeting your vision with a clear structure: a detailed plan, an organized execution, and systems for productivity. You are here to be of service and will likely be called into the healing arts. But steer clear of martyrdom.

North Node in Pisces, South Node in Virgo: Build your faith in the universe and find comfort in knowing that you can trust the flow of life. Your spiritual practices hold the key to personal fulfillment and soul satisfaction. Stay mindful of perfectionistic tendencies. You have astute healing capacities and a service-driven soul. Just make sure you make time for you. Whenever possible, lean into music, art, and self-expression.

Monthly Lunar Rituals

In a typical month (some months are atypical) there are two main lunar events: a new moon and a full moon.

A new moon is the perfect time to set intentions to realize your desires. You can do that by clearly writing out an intention for that lunar cycle and actively working with it through the entire lunar cycle. Ideally, your intention will align with the sign that the new moon occurs in. (In chapter 15, I provide you with a new moon ritual.)

Full moons are a time to cultivate your power. The full moon is also a time of the month when your intuition may feel heightened and your energy may feel "different." How a full moon affects you is specific to you.

Full Moon Ritual

Rituals are like recipes: the best ones have been honed over time. Treat the following full-moon ritual as a jumping-off point, not a final destination. This one connects you to the elements and helps you balance the earth, air, fire, and water within.

First, set the tone for your ritual. This begins with assessing your physical space and how it feels to you. Is it clean? Is it cluttered? Do what you can to make your space feel like a conduit for transformation.

While cleaning, play music that feels like a match for the energy you wish to call in.

Before you do your ritual, take a *cosmic bath.* (If you prefer showers, they work just the same, but with a shower use a salt scrub instead of bath salts.) Draw your bath, adding one to two cups of Epsom salts and a few drops of your favorite essential oil if you use them. I generally suggest lavender or eucalyptus, but any will do, and it's your preference. You may also want to add a few flowers to your bathwater, or anything that evokes a sense of inspiring beauty.

Soak in the bathtub for twenty minutes. Imagine the salts removing anything that is less than divine as your skin absorbs the magnesium.

When you get out of the bath, nourish your body with a healing oil, like sesame or jojoba. As you massage your body, intentionally visualize what you wish to call into your life.

After applying the oil, dress yourself in an outfit that feels special to you. This can be your favorite pair of pajamas, a party dress, or simply whatever you feel comfortable in.

Next, go to a place in your house where you can meditate, preferably by an altar. You'll want a candle, incense, pen, paper, and a lighter or match. Take a moment to center yourself and then light your incense and candle.

Once you've lit your incense, connect with the elements:

- Honor the element of *air* by connecting with your breath. Inhale and exhale deeply.
- Honor the element of *fire* by connecting with your desire. Visualize your desire for your health and your life. Conjure as much passion for yourself as you can.

- Honor the element of *water* by connecting with your intuition. Listen to the quiet voice within. What is she whispering in your ear or communicating to you through your feelings? Take a moment to write down what you're hearing. If journaling works better for you, journal on this question: *What is my truth right now?*
- Honor the element of *earth* by connecting with your body. How does she feel? What does she need?
- Now, go outside, and if the night is clear, stand in the moonlight. Take at least five minutes meditating on the moon, and bathing in her light. You can do so with your eyes open or closed, whatever feels right to you. Say a prayer or repeat an affirmation. Let yourself become absorbed in the moment, connecting to the light of the moon and your inner power. You can do so with your eyes open or closed, but the idea is to connect with the moon's light, when that's possible, and simultaneously with your personal power. Say a prayer or repeat an affirmation that you are working on.

Once you feel complete, come back in and return to your altar and/ or candle. Take a moment to integrate the experience. Then, thank yourself, the Earth, and the moon. Extinguish the candle and bring your ritual to a close.

CHAPTER 6

The Sun Sign

Be Who You Are

J ust be yourself."

We hear this constantly, but what does it actually mean? While often left undefined, the underlying promise of this saying is clear: when we navigate life as our "true" selves, we thrive in every way—physically, emotionally, spiritually, financially, in relationships, and within communities.

Sounds lovely, doesn't it?

In astrology, your natal sun sign acts as a gateway to knowing your authentic self. It's the essence of how you animate your daytime energy. We'll go through each sun sign in this chapter, but first, let's look at what being yourself means in the context of achieving cosmic health.

Being Your (Ever-Changing, Multifaceted) Self

Author and psychologist David Schnarch teaches the importance of having a solid flexible self (a term he trademarked). When it comes to achieving a solid flexible self, it's essential to move away from sourcing validation from others and instead build our capacity to self-validate. When we self-validate, we no longer need to sculpt a persona to be liked.

Instead of looking to others for acceptance, we generate self-acceptance from within.

In doing so, we strive to be known, not validated.[1] The goal of authenticity, then, is to experience the freedom that comes from feeling coherent and aligned with our truth.

But again, we need to define what that means—in the context of cosmic health but also in terms of our everyday lives and the many different roles we play. Plus, can we truly be ourselves at all times, and in all circumstances? And how can we be ourselves when we're continuously transforming and evolving?

I had a long and enlightening conversation with a client of mine on these very topics. As a married mother and a corporate lawyer with a deep connection to spiritual practices rooted in her ancestry, Ana, an Afro-Latina woman, embodies both the promise and paradox of being yourself.

With her natal sun in Leo, she is innately pulled toward self-expression. For her, being her true self has meant embracing the many different parts and pieces of herself. Since she no longer feels a need to align with just one part of herself—corporate professional or spiritual seeker or mother or wife—Ana does not feel the pressure to compartmentalize herself. Being her corporate self is just as real and true as being her spiritual seeker self, and so on.

This wasn't always so easy for her, though. Growing up in the US as a Black woman whose family had emigrated from Brazil made it hard for her to "be herself." Not easily fitting into any one group, she was left to grapple with many nuances as they related to her race and identity. When she set out to reclaim a connection to her Afro-Latina ancestry, she struggled, toggling between many different aspects of her identity at once: Black American, South American with Indigenous ancestral roots, a high-performing college student at a predominantly white university, and a soon-to-be lawyer.

While challenging, over the years she learned that by accepting herself as a multifaceted and ever-evolving being, she can move gracefully between the different parts of herself and the roles she plays without sacrificing her personal truth or understanding of who she is. That's because doing so doesn't involve self-betrayal.

Now, as a woman in midlife, Ana continues to evolve. As she does, her nuanced understanding of who she is remains flexible and fluid. She welcomes her ever-evolving spiritual growth with grace and humility, without compromising her truth or sincerity. This is what I'm referring to when I talk about becoming more authentic in ourselves and our lives. The reality is, few of us can be every part of ourselves all the time, and with all people. That's because our lives, like our astrology charts, have many aspects. We can honor them all yet also accept that the different parts ebb and flow continuously.

Understanding Your Sun Sign

In the previous chapter, we looked at how your natal moon sign highlights your deeper emotional needs. Your natal sun sign, which represents your core identity, and your overall disposition, deepens your understanding of yourself. It is your creative energy, who you are and how you get things done.

Your sun sign is the zodiacal sign the sun traveled through at the time of your birth. Just as your moon sign provides insight into a vast range of deeper emotional needs and desires, your sun sign gives you an expansive framework to work with as you grow and evolve. Knowing the ins and outs of your sun sign also highlights the nuances of your overall life path as well as your journey toward health and genuine, fulfilling self-expression.

As with your natal moon sign, you may relate to most if not all of the characteristics of your sun sign — or not. Either response is okay. While indicative of your core archetype, and important for learning how to be yourself, your sun sign doesn't define the totality of who you are.

The hallmark qualities and energies of each sun sign include light and dark aspects. They're neither good nor bad, but they can be strengths or weaknesses, depending on the context. For instance, Pisces is considered a highly intuitive sign. An archetype for Pisces is the healer. The light side, the strength here, is that a Pisces can experience deep empathy and compassion for others. The other side, or weakness, is that a Pisces may become too emotionally invested in other people's lives and play the role of the victim or martyr as a result.

The more you learn about what makes you uniquely you, the more adept you'll become at identifying when certain traits are helpful, or not. You'll also be able to amplify your strengths while being mindful and compassionate about your challenges, which is essential to your emotional well-being and also your physical health.

Loving *All* of Who You Are

As a thirty-eight-year-old Australian living in Sydney and running a massively successful multimillion-dollar business, Shelly was a quintessential hardworking Capricorn. Her drive to be the best and maintain her authority had taken her far, but it was also taking a toll on her health and her life.

Physically and emotionally depleted, Shelly felt disembodied and overwhelmed by a deep sense of failure around her fraying marriage and family life. Ashamed of her inability to balance work, family, and health, she was filled with self-loathing.

Truthfully, she was miserable. As a Capricorn, she believed self-care was a waste of time. However, she felt trapped by her business and knew that she needed to make a change.

Through our coaching, she realized she was overworking to avoid intimacy with herself and, consequently, her family — a pattern she learned from her dad. He taught her that success meant sacrifice. To him being worthy required grinding day in and day out, without ever relenting or adequately resting.

Soon, she began to schedule more frequent vacations, which created the time she needed to repair her relationship with her partner and connect with her daughter. Working less, she naturally began to sleep better, exercise more, and finally relax.

Now she enjoys time parenting and connecting with her partner without sacrificing her ambition. She's excited about creating a new business, but she's no longer trying to "escape" her life by overworking. Instead, she's enjoying being in the life she's created wholeheartedly.

Understanding her sun sign allowed her to tap into her strengths, name her weaknesses, and accept both as part of who she is. This self-compassion inspired her to rewrite a new definition of success.

Some clients resist the idea of self-compassion, worried that being "soft" on themselves will lead to complacency and resigned acceptance of the status quo. In fact, the opposite is true—when we can accept and love all of ourselves, we can transform what's no longer working. I use this practice in my daily life. Whenever I judge or criticize myself, I try to meet that voice with love, tenderness, and gentleness. Through this softer filter, I can then notice any decisions and behaviors that I'd like to change.

As you learn more about your sun sign's strengths and weaknesses, your capacity for self-love and self-compassion will be challenged. That's okay! Sitting with those difficult emotions without sacrificing self-compassion is one of the most important forms of self-care you will ever practice. While it may not qualify as feel-good self-care, it is hugely important for your emotional well-being, and therefore, your overall health and happiness.

ON ANY REDUNDANCY IN YOUR CHART

If the same sign repeats in your moon, sun, and/or rising (ascendant), take the sign's descriptions to heart. If, for instance, your natal sun and moon signs are both Taurus, your natal sun and moon sign descriptions may seem repetitive. Rather than disregarding one or the other, use that redundancy as an opportunity to notice how, say, your connection to the earth and affinity for comfort play out in your internal experience (through your moon sign) and in your sense of self and vitality (through your sun sign).

Your Sun Sign and Self-Care

Self-care brings us back to center and helps to bolster resilience by providing much-needed respite in an otherwise harried life. It's a form of replenishment in our depletion-centric world.

Self-care is sometimes seen as indulgent, but taking care of your needs is a basic necessity. If you skimp on self-care, you compromise one of the most important aspects of life: your dignity. According to Dr. Donna Hicks, author of the bestselling book *Dignity: The Essential Role It Plays in Resolving Conflict*, dignity means respecting your inherent value and worth.[2] You foster dignity through acknowledgment; feeling seen, heard, witnessed, included; and having a sense of belonging and community as well as a healthy sense of independence. You honor your dignity by seeking to understand yourself and others. Self-care is one important way to do that. It's an essential acknowledgment of your right to exist, to take up space and time in your life and your calendar.

In the words of feminist theologian Meggan Watterson, "Worth is not earned, it's claimed."[3] Worthiness isn't granted; it's revealed and retrieved. Regardless of your body size, occupation, wild professional success (or lack thereof), relationship status, or any other benchmark, you are dignified. You are worthy.

Just as your sun sign reveals how you animate your life-force energy, it also reveals your unique needs and suggests ways to fulfill them.

The Sun in Your Natal Chart: Putting It to Work for You

The following is an overview of all twelve sun signs. In each one I break down the core attributes of that sign as well as the strengths and challenges associated with that sign. Consider this another piece of your natal chart puzzle, all of which, when combined, will point you toward powerful ways to increase your baseline level of health and well-being.

WHAT IF YOU WERE BORN ON A DAY WHEN THE SUN CHANGED SIGNS, AKA A SIGN CUSP?

I have a dear friend who, had he been born five minutes earlier, would have had an entirely different natal sun sign. Yet he was born when he was born, and is indeed a Pisces, not an Aquarius. Since any zodiac sign encompasses thirty degrees, you can be born at a late degree of one sign or an early degree of another, but not both. The dates for the sun signs below are estimated. If you are born on a cusp, calculating your chart is essential to knowing your sun sign.

♈ ARIES
(MARCH 21–APRIL 19)

Pioneer. Director. Athlete.

Symbol: Ram
Element: Fire
Ruling Planet: Mars
Mode: Cardinal

Your Strengths

As an Aries, you are a born boss, the initiator who can spot the ebb of patriarchal traditions and the flow of soon-to-be trends — and deliver the firepower to bring an idea into reality. Because of this, you are highly motivated and capable of leading. You're a pioneer, whether you think of yourself that way or not. As a cardinal fire sign of action, growth, and new beginnings, you know what you want. With your insatiable appetite for movement, it won't take long to climb any mountain you set your sights on. Create space in your life to zero in on your exact desire and channel that ferocity to make it happen. You're better at delegating than you know, so be sure to distribute your workload accordingly.

Your Challenges

As an innovator, you're here to weave new impressions into the world and change the way we function. Let's be real: everyone may not get on board right away. While it may be irritating when others can't keep up with your pace, recognize this as a part of life. Learning how to slow down is essential for you. Your assertive nature can come across as both energizing and domineering. Pay close attention to avoid alienating people by being overly pushy and aggressive. Embrace discipline and beware of your rebellious tendencies, which can cause you to impulsively burn bridges. You are here this lifetime to learn tenacity and relentless devotion.

Your Self-Care

With Mars as your ruling planet, you may love speed, although perhaps too much at times. You want what you want, like, yesterday. Learning how to be patient with challenges, and the sometimes *very* slow timeline it takes to manifest the results you seek, is where the magic happens. To feel fresh and inspired, use a mindfulness practice that helps you be in the moment, and take plenty of time for rest. While quitting can be a way of self-honoring—not everything you start will be finished   giving up too soon leads you down the road of a lot of false starts. Make a commitment and stick with it, especially with goals that fuel your ambition, which is key to staying passionate and healthy. Stay mindful of anger as it can sometimes block grief. Give yourself the time you need to cry and process pain. Lucky for you, your ruling planet, Mars, only goes retrograde once every two years, but when he does, it's essential for you to use that time to recalibrate your ambition and rethink your goals.

Your Physical Health

Your constitution requires ample physical movement and plenty of whole foods, like leafy greens and high-quality proteins. Deep breathing will also help you to release CO_2, which supports an acid–alkaline balance, as well as temper your sense of urgency. Pay attention to your sinuses, head, and eyes, particularly if you're prone to headaches and migraines. Using a neti pot regularly is a simple way to keep your sinuses clear. Since your ruling planet, Mars, governs muscles, healing practices that move energy through your neuromuscular system often offer the immediate relief you crave. For example, acupuncture, body-centered psychotherapy, and massage help you to metabolize the intense feelings that sometimes arise. Kickboxing, running, spinning, and other cardio activities refresh and inspire you, although it's important not to overdo it, which will put added stress on your adrenal glands, a contraindication. The key to satisfying success is to stay in alignment with your body's needs, which means taking your exercise to your edge but no further. Build in time to relax and recover from huge spurts of energy.

♉ TAURUS
(APRIL 20–MAY 20)
Epicurean. Gardener. Aphrodite.

Symbol: Bull
Element: Earth
Ruling Planet: Venus
Mode: Fixed

Your Strengths

As a Taurus, you are tough, loyal, and steadfast. Own your independence and choose projects wisely, because once you start, you won't stop until everything is done, and done well. With a gentle, feel-good presence, you provide stability with a creative twist; your keen sense of beauty and sensuality makes you an able nurturer. You excel at cultivating resources and abiding rhythms. As the first fixed sign and earth sign in the zodiac, Taurus finds comfort and pleasure in the material realm. Motivate yourself by indulging your senses—put your bare feet to the ground and consciously connect with Gaia. Own your extremely refined sensibility by holding tight to your standards. You raise the bar for others.

Your Challenges

Your connection to the earth as well as earthly delights, like great food, pleasure, and even a little luxury, are important for you to feel grounded and balanced. Yet you can use physical pleasure to avoid facing tough problems. Transcend the material by getting out of your comfort zone; your love of life should help you sink deeper into your spiritual purpose, not distance you from it. Curb overindulgence and rigidity. Adding variety to your life amplifies your resilience. Learn to reframe narratives, challenge your beliefs, and understand different perspectives.

Your Self-Care

You are naturally capable of self-nurturing, especially with Venus as your ruling planet. Your tenacious commitment means you don't ever quit, relent, or give up hope. Leverage these positive traits to your advantage. Typically gentle and hardworking, you truly enjoy being a part of the world. However, your ideal pace is unhurried, and you can dig in your heels when you're pushed too hard, too soon. This leads you to push back, which can create an argumentative atmosphere. Stay mindful of your triggers. Conscientious, responsible care is the bedrock of great work, yet don't forget, self-care means trying new things and expanding your horizon. Practice getting more comfortable with uncertainty. Lucky for you, your ruling planet, Venus, only goes retrograde once every eighteen months, but when she does, it's essential for you to use that time to recalibrate your inner needs.

Your Physical Health

Taurus rules the throat and connects your head to the base of your spine, bridging your mind and your body. The throat also connects to the diaphragm and pelvic floor, so using your breath is a way to access your innate power and deeper relaxation. Similarly, the throat houses your vocal cords. So owning your voice and speaking your truth is medicinal for you. Belt out songs whenever you can. Caring for your thyroid is essential too. Ironically, this means taking excellent care of your gut, which helps prevent autoimmune conditions. Watch your estrogen levels, and do your best to avoid endocrine-disrupting chemicals. Avoid overindulging in sweets, alcohol, and pleasure-based eating, and find an exercise routine that works for you. Remember, body size is not a measure of health. Practice loving yourself *exactly* as you are. Your ruling planet, Venus, makes a sense of touch extra special for you, so self-massage is really healing!

♊ GEMINI
(MAY 21–JUNE 20)

Networker. Teacher. Writer.

Symbol: Twins
Element: Air
Ruling Planet: Mercury
Mode: Mutable

Your Strengths

Ideas and creativity are brewing inside you, and you can't wait to bring them to fruition. Known for your multifaceted wit, you are high-energy and don magician-like qualities to manifest at record speed. As an air sign ruled by the messenger Mercury, your quick-witted, social, communicative nature allows you to meet new friends and acquaintances easily. You make great things happen by connecting people and ideas in unique ways. Keenly observational, you stay sharp and in the know. An adept and collaborative leader, you are also an able writer and communicator.

Your Challenges

As a mutable air sign, you always have a million thoughts running through your mind. You could research and daydream forever, but are your ideas meant to stay there? It's crucial to discern what to focus on *next*—and commit to it. Gemini being one of the most noncommittal signs of the zodiac, tempering your desire to start, stop, and start again may feel harder than turning water into wine. But I promise, you can create consistency. With so many interests, you may get a bad rap for being fickle—here today, gone tomorrow. Also, when operating from your shadow, you can be a deleterious gossip. Be as trustworthy as the secrets you can keep.

Your Self-Care

The key to soulful, satisfying self-care is to make sure your ideas don't get clotted up inside you. A regular writing or journaling practice will do you wonders. You may overindulge your extroverted side, so be aware of your tendency to run yourself ragged. Consciously slow down by under-scheduling yourself by 20 percent. Keeping open space in your calendar will temper the resentment that comes from saying yes to *everything* and then regretting it later or bailing at the last minute. Know your red flags—mood swings, anxiety, and acute depression—and take necessary personal time, including social media and digital detoxes, which will help calm the mind and nervous system too. Since you are ruled by Mercury, pay attention to his retrograde cycles, which happen three to four times every year. These times are meant to support you by allowing you to integrate the lessons you are learning. Use them as sacred times throughout the year.

Your Physical Health

Gemini rules the shoulders, arms, hands, and lungs, while Mercury, your ruling planet, rules the nervous system, making meditation and yogic breathing, also known as pranayama, medicinal for you. They will help you to manage anxiety, a common Gemini issue, and focus. This means working to develop a strong mind–body connection is critical for you. Understanding your body's needs helps you stay grounded. Try developing and sticking to a routine; learning to do the same thing at the same time every day grounds your body and allows you to eat for nourishment, move for energy, and sleep for peace. However unnatural it may feel at first, routine is everything for you. When it comes to physical movement, you do best with something that has an upbeat tempo: think hiking, a mild jog, shooting hoops, Hula-Hooping, or dancing.

♋ CANCER
(JUNE 21–JULY 22)
Empress. Breadwinner. Nurturer.

Symbol: Crab
Element: Water
Ruling Planet: Moon
Mode: Cardinal

Your Strengths

As a cardinal water sign that's associated with traditions of the distant past, you're a natural gardener of the soil and the soul. Born under one of the most nurturing signs of the zodiac, you have a knack for helping loved ones feel safe and secure that is nearly unparalleled. Yet your presence is steeped in the sacred, which also makes you a fierce protector — especially when those you love feel threatened. That feeds your propensity to create security in your life. You're adept at cultivating your assets, both psychological strengths and material well-being. Doing just that allows you to boldly pursue whatever is on your horizon, or the horizons of loved ones, with peace of mind. Build your nest egg and simultaneously enjoy nesting in your home too.

Your Challenges

Emotional waters run deep with the fourth sign of the zodiac, and for good reason. This sign is most susceptible to carrying other people's burdens and heartbreaks. Those around you sense your innate power to soothe, so they may unintentionally (or intentionally) pour their pain into your psyche. While they may feel better, you'll eventually find yourself dragging under others' hefty emotional weight. Because of this—and the fact that you are ruled by the moon, which changes signs faster than any other planet—you can come across as moody, even crabby. Slowing down and getting grounded brings you back to your center and helps you source power from within.

Your Self-Care

Prone to giving and nurturing, your natural warmth and generosity bring people closer together. However, sometimes we serve those we love best by saying no so that they can fulfill their own soul growth. More than most other signs, it's important for you to establish and maintain healthy boundaries. While taking care of those around you may come easily, your true power lies in discernment. Not all emotion is yours to hold, and the sooner you accept that, the sooner you can step into your own true emotional current. Tending to emotional pain from your past and transgenerational trauma, and healing family dynamics, is critical for you. As is working with the moon's phases.

Your Physical Health

Cancer correlates with the chest and breast—how you give and receive nurturing. Yet learning how to get things "off your chest" means getting comfortable with discomfort. Your body functions like a natural record keeper, storing memories and stories from long ago. Mindfully connecting to emotional pain helps you move through it, but also learning how to physically release it from your body helps you experience emotional catharsis. Stagnancy in your body creates stagnancy in your life. When this happens, you experience bouts of insomnia, get stuck in ruminative thinking, and are prone to anxiety. Stretching, yoga, working with the fascial system, and somatic therapies that tend to address trauma in the body are really important to you. Spending time on, or near, water always brings you back to center. The same is true of music, which, ideally, you listen to daily. Also, observing the impact of your ruling planet, the moon, as it orbits around Earth, forming different positions to the sun and celestial bodies, will help you track and leverage your physiological and biological rhythms.

♌ LEO
(JULY 23–AUGUST 22)
Sovereign. Motivator. Leader.

Symbol: Lion
Element: Fire
Ruling Planet: Sun
Mode: Fixed

Your Strengths

Ruled by the sun and born under the fifth sign of the zodiac, Leo *must* experience life from a place of creativity, self-expression, generosity, and fun. As fixed fire, you represent pure potential—the shaky breath an actor takes before marching on stage, the first spark of a bonfire in the woods. People are drawn to your innate warmth and a golden quality that makes them feel that you've got everything handled. This ability to help people feel safe and accepted makes you a lion-hearted leader. You're comfortable being center stage, although you may not always seek it out. Naturally playful, confident, generous, and bold, Leos, as influencers, can engage others and help them find their own shine too.

Your Challenges

While you may garner a fair amount of attention and love, receiving it is not always comfortable. By learning to shift attention onto others, you can mitigate that discomfort and engage your innate generosity too. If you're comfortable at the center of attention, fine-tune your self-reflection. As a fixed fire sign, stepping down may prove especially challenging. You may be attracted to drama, but you're better served by channeling your energy into creative pursuits. Develop an intuitive practice—art, journaling, writing, or another mode of creative self-expression—to release tension and discern where your leadership skills are most needed. Approach conflict with an open heart and mindful listening, and let your intuitive nature lead.

Your Self-Care

Leo is all about taking a stand, no matter how much courage it requires. Do what you must to stay brave. But watch out for your ego, Leo. You aren't always right. If you have a lot of Leo energy in your natal chart, you are wired a little differently. As a living, breathing representation of pure potential, you need to metaphorically live from your center—your heart. That means the avid pursuit of what you love and ample doses of fun. Yet your emotional health requires you to learn to love yourself with your vulnerabilities. Work on developing compassion for the parts of you that you find less desirable. Once you can integrate the light *and* the dark, and the lessons of each, you can become the powerful, sovereign leader you were meant to be. As a natural giver, you can over-give...and end up depleted. Taking time to fill your own tank is key.

Your Physical Health

Leo is ruled by the sun, so spending time outdoors, under the sun, is essential for you. Expose yourself to natural daylight early in the morning. This helps to suppress melatonin and stimulates a healthy hormonal response to fuel your daytime energy. Remember your well-being is intertwined with Earth's rotation and revolution around the sun, through the rhythms of your body. To maximize this connection, take ample vacations to warm locations. Playing nourishes your body and helps you de-escalate from stress. Living seasonally is especially important to you. As the sun changes signs, you change too. So pay attention to the various qualities of the zodiacal year, and leverage their potential month by month. When you unfurl the tension in your back, your lion heart naturally shines.

♍ VIRGO
(AUGUST 23–SEPTEMBER 22)

Mentor. Engineer. Editor.

Symbol: Virgin
Element: Earth
Ruling Planet: Mercury
Mode: Mutable

Your Strengths

I lovingly refer to you, Virgo, with your refined sense of precision, as the "protector of purity." As the responsible, service-oriented editor of the zodiac, you bring order to excess and abundance. While the "neat freak" stereotype persists, you aren't always perfectly organized. When you take on a project, you give it your all, but that sometimes means letting go of other responsibilities, including cleaning. You desire to make a positive impact in the world through service and tend to be productive and humble in your work, putting foolproof systems in place to get things done. While the rest of us are still figuring out what to eat for breakfast, you can process data, develop routines, and build structures that keep everything in order. Your attention span and penchant for details are considerable, but it's your sense of responsibility that makes you stand apart. In that minuscule moment when most of us would throw in the towel, your fortitude pushes you onward.

Your Challenges

While you excel at categorizing and organizing, you are also prone to overthinking. People and situations that you can't easily sort are likely to gnaw at you. You'll pick at the edges of something until you can get it to fit in your box. This can create anxiety and result in perfectionist behavior. With a tendency to pack your life full — of details, supporting others, and your work — you are always so, so busy. Yet being that busy doesn't leave enough time for you. Learn to underschedule yourself so you can accommodate your own needs. This doesn't mean being less caring. It means not glorifying busyness. Dare I even say it?! Take a vacation!

Your Self-Care

Remember that sometimes it's okay to let go of the details. Release the need for perfection and find ways to be calm in the mess. Not everything will be picture-perfect. Developing a self-care practice like meditation can bring you back to the present moment and create a sense of coherence in your body. Remember that a strong self-care ritual helps you be in service to others. Your sensitive nature needs alone time — it balances you out. Steer clear of pitfalls like rumination and negative thinking that can spiral out of control, giving way to anxiety. This is a product of overthinking.

Your Physical Health

While you are very concerned about the health of the people and world around you, remember that self-care aids you to be of service to others. Your sensitive nature requires consistent loving care. Virgo rules your abdomen, which houses many of the organs that participate in the digestive process. The intestines (particularly the small intestine), digestive enzymes, diaphragm, liver, stomach, and nervous system in the gut — collectively referred to as your enteric nervous system — all work together so you can assimilate and eliminate nutrition and waste. The enteric nervous system is called the "second brain," which is why trusting your gut is just as important as your ability to arrive at a decision analytically. Pay attention to it by avoiding foods that throw you and your blood sugar out of balance. Just as important is to eat mindfully. Your digestion starts in your mouth, so learning to eat slower and chew your food is helpful. Like Gemini, the ruling planet of your sun sign, Mercury, goes retrograde three to four times a year, allowing you sacred times throughout the year to recalibrate and reassess your goals. Keep those as sacred timeframes when you pay even closer attention to your health.

♎ LIBRA
(SEPTEMBER 23–OCTOBER 22)
Artist. Advocate. Liberator.

Symbol: Scales
Element: Air
Ruling Planet: Venus
Mode: Cardinal

Your Strengths

As the seventh sign of the zodiac, the start of Libra season marks the center of the astrological calendar, which is exactly how you prefer it. As a cardinal air sign, you're rarely short on acquaintances or topics of conversation, but you're at your best when you can connect to others at their core. Ruled by Venus, you are drawn to art, beauty, culture, and sophistication. Your journey to deeper self-knowledge happens through your relationships. It may seem paradoxical to find yourself through others, but in the words of psychologist Carl Rogers, "what's most personal is most universal." A natural keeper of the peace, you care deeply about justice and balance — not just getting the work done but doing so in harmony with others, your environment, and the world around you. Your healing, judicious presence helps you excel at making things happen. You are brilliant at building community and cultivating friendships.

Your Challenges

People-pleasing and passive-aggressive behavior come easily to you, as a conflict-averse sign, and you may self-sacrifice to keep the peace. For you, the grass is always green on both sides of the fence. Your ability to cut through the BS and see the pure potential in any situation means that often you see what something *could* be instead of what it truly is. Sometimes the grass isn't even grass... it's just mud. While it's easy to see the best in others and win over friends with your social charm, you'll first need to begin a loving relationship with yourself. Dress up and take yourself out to dinner. Learn to say no and do less. Take a step back from always organizing and leading. Otherwise, you risk becoming resentful and burning out, especially when overcommitted. When you know what matters most to you, it's easy to make decisions around your relationships that align with your values.

Your Self-Care

The high value you place on fairness and harmony can make confronting conflict and owning darker emotions especially challenging. How can you make confrontation less intimidating? Develop emotional resilience by learning how to accept, feel, and express anger without aggression. Learn that it is okay to disappoint others. Acknowledge and accept your people-pleasing tendencies, and then work on prioritizing yourself as much as others. Like Taurus, the ruling planet of your sun sign, Venus, makes indulging in art a critical piece of your emotional and spiritual health. Remember, Venus only goes retrograde once every eighteen months. Those are extremely special times for you to integrate your shadow and emerge in your strength.

Your Physical Health

Letting go of what's not working and accentuating what is working is essential to restoring your equilibrium. Pay special attention to your kidneys and lower back, as well as your body's ability to rid itself of waste. You can bend over backwards to please others, which can leave you feeling overextended and in pain. If you find yourself propping up your energy or spirits with caffeine or sugar, take a day off and rest. Remember, Venus also relates to the throat, and there's a connection between the throat and your pelvic floor. Using your voice helps you to access your erotic nature. Speaking your mind, and even singing, allows you to feel more embodied and free.

♏ SCORPIO
(OCTOBER 23–NOVEMBER 21)
Sorceress. Therapist. Investigator.

Symbol: Scorpion
Element: Water
Ruling Planets: Pluto and Mars
Mode: Fixed

Your Strengths

The warning growl of a wolf protecting her den. The mechanism behind magic. Death. Rebirth. This is the Scorpio essence in action. There's no denying your intensity, but you're well prepared to handle the ride. As a water sign, you're adept at reading emotional energy and metaphysical undercurrents, which makes your sense of timing impeccable. You know exactly when to strike on closing that deal, even if external evidence suggests otherwise. Your fierce ambition and independence often put you in a place of power—and you're determined to become the best. Dedicated to profound truth and authenticity, you waste no time on the superficial. You thrive when digging deep and dealing with complicated ideas, emotions, and secrets.

Your Challenges

Scorpio gets a bad rap for heralding chaos, but you shouldn't be blamed for being a harbinger of anarchy. Ruled by aggressive Mars and mysterious Pluto, it's no wonder that a certain level of discomfort follows you. In reality, your job is to help people cut ties with anything that isn't to their highest benefit. Prone to protect yourself, you can come across as guarded. Intimacy softens you, lights you up, and expands your sense of abundance. Chaos, after all, is the void that preceded all creation. Embracing the cyclical power of birth–death–rebirth allows you to resurrect as your strongest self. But please stay mindful of your tendencies to want to feel safe by exercising control. Learning how to "be" is essential for you.

Your Self-Care

As the natural introvert of the zodiac, you need a lot of alone time to rejuvenate. Time spent turning inward allows you to realize your ability to transform ruins into blooms. Stay aware of your own faults so you can then lovingly help others see their own. You tend to have secrets, so opening up and letting go is critical for you. Engage in cathartic activities that help you to release energy and emotion. Tame jealousy with a spiritual practice. Be mindful of your fixed nature. Your highly developed intuition comes from your soul's relentless urge to get to the truth. You aren't into sugarcoating, mostly because you know that playing nice serves no one. Unafraid of what you'll uncover when you start digging, you figure you'll at least know the truth before it can damage your sensitive soul.

Your Physical Health

Scorpio rules the pelvic region, including parts of the birthing process as well as the process of dying. So tending to your menstrual cycle or reproductive organs remains essential for you. It's especially important for you to have a healthy sex life. Even if you don't have a partner, self-pleasure provides a vital connection to yourself. Pluto, Scorpio's ruling planet, governs the body's metabolic powers and its process of elimination. Making sure you are taking regular poops assists you in staying healthy. My medical astrology teacher, Rebecca Gordon, talks about how the "sacrum," which is composed of the five fused bones at the base of the spine, comes from the Latin *os sacrum*, which means "sacred."[4] Since the modern ruler of your sun sign is Pluto, pay close attention to his retrograde cycles, which happen every year for approximately five months. During that time you are called to tend to your health by integrating your shadow and letting go of all that no longer serves you.

↗ SAGITTARIUS
(NOVEMBER 22–DECEMBER 21)
Bon Vivant. Teacher. Truth Seeker.

Symbol: Archer
Element: Fire
Ruling Planet: Jupiter
Mode: Mutable

Your Strengths

If you've ever had an insatiable urge to meander down a winding trail with no idea where it ends, your Sagittarius spirit is shining bright. Your intuitive wandering may take you to an open-air market in Marrakech or cause you to hop on an airplane with only the clothes on your back. Ruled by optimistic and expansive Jupiter, you abhor rules and adore independence, adventure, travel, and philosophy. You live to explore, grow, and attain the unattainable—and then show others how to do the same. Born under the ninth sign of the zodiac, you have an unwaveringly positive outlook that brings you luck. As the sign of the archer, you are deeply motivated to aim at your desire and hit it dead center. You say whatever is on your mind. Blessed with the ability to see the whole picture, you can keep your eyes on the prize without getting distracted by shiny trinkets and toxic relationships on your way to the top. Half the fun is how you get there, right?

Your Challenges

As a fire sign, you're on an eternal quest for the truth, yet as a Sag, sometimes you are a bit too blunt with others. (Not everyone is ready for your honesty.) Because you need to express yourself without boundaries, you must do things alone and with total authority. Spend time writing, doing art, researching, exploring mindfulness, or any activity that lets you self-express and follow your instincts unflinchingly. You don't like it when things feel boring, have too many rules, or put you in a box, so make a point of seeking out adventure, even if that means taking a different route to work. Schedule regular mini-adventures, or book that once-in-a-lifetime cross-continental trip. If you can't take off, take a winding detour through the library to pick up a book you usually wouldn't, meet up with new friends at that dive bar you've meant to check out, or try a new restaurant. You are philosophical by nature, but remember, just because you believe something doesn't mean everyone else has to agree. Your ruling planet, Jupiter, who amplifies growth, goes retrograde each year for roughly four months. During this time, you may feel even more curious about what lights you and how you can live with more enthusiasm.

Your Self-Care

To reach your potential, you need to embrace a wee bit of discipline, which isn't your favorite word. You love to go big, which means indulging gratuitously in what you desire. But more isn't always better. Learning your limits allows you to thrive, especially with things that feel good in the moment, but leave you depleted. (Think sugar, alcohol, and frivolously spending your time on things that provide no genuine nourishment.) When stuck, ponder the core concept that informs who you are, how you live, and what you desire to create. More than most, it helps to spend time with your people — those who welcome all of you, your sense of humor, your contagious spirit, and your self-expression, and who don't shame your authenticity. Ask lots of questions and listen to the answers, especially the ones that your body provides. When you develop an intuitive way of knowing what you need, you always have a compass guiding you precisely where you need to go next.

Your Potential

Freedom is vital to you, so choose exercises that complement your naturally rebellious nature. Think hip-hop dance, belly dancing, drumming, and even pole dancing. When a Sagittarius gets lazy, it's all too easy to lose vitality and feel depressed, which makes tending to your physical health critical to your mental well-being. Engaging in mindfulness and developing an authentic connection to your spiritual purpose helps you to feel strong. For you, there's nothing more healing than wholehearted laugh-until-you-cry fun. Hysterical movies, comedy clubs, and even laughter yoga offer you critical nourishment. Push back on normative beauty standards and celebrate your body exactly as she is. Yes, you can strive to feel more fit, but do so because it feels good, not because you want to win others' approval or pander to patriarchal standards. Sagittarius rules the thighs and hips—the lower parts of the body that allow you to travel—so yoga's pigeon pose and other hip openers can also help you. Your ruling planet, Jupiter, corresponds with the liver and pituitary gland. Be sure that your diet includes plenty of water, high-quality proteins, healthy fats, and lots of leafy greens. Stay mindful of refined foods, eat a blood-sugar balanced diet, and take care of your HPA axis by sleeping well at night.

♑ CAPRICORN
(DECEMBER 22–JANUARY 19)
Expert. Strategist. Executive.

Symbol: Sea Goat
Element: Earth
Ruling Planet: Saturn
Mode: Cardinal

Your Strengths

As a Capricorn, you embody the ability to manifest not only a seat at the table but an entire institution. Ruled by authoritarian Saturn, you aren't one to take responsibilities lightly. Capricorns are here to learn what it means to fulfill their responsibilities, even when—especially when—the process requires inordinate amounts of patience, perseverance, and hard work. Things may not always come easily, but they always come when you commit. Tenacious like no other, you're inspired to break away from indulgence in order to defy the odds and become the most extraordinary version of yourself. Given your serious and practical side, your business savvy is on point. With a keen sense of how much hustling it takes to bring something into being, you naturally respect what is already in place. Instead of burning down existing foundations, why not build upon what's already there and change it from the inside out?

Your Challenges

Just because you don't wear your heart on your sleeve doesn't mean you don't feel deeply. In fact, your impeccable sense of duty pushes you to explore your intuition and soul wisdom. If you're truly going to be your best, you have to develop *all* of you. When you receive an intuitive hit, you tend to take it seriously. Sometimes you allow things to become harder than they need to be. Don't let your desire to succeed keep you from letting go when it's called for! Your tendency to work hard can lead to an absence of play. Remember to stop and find ease and wonder in the amazing things you do.

Your Self-Care

To reach your highest potential, you must embrace the paradox of practical wisdom. You're here to show others what it means to achieve by mastering the less flashy things of life—routines, habits, and structure. While you enjoy your accomplishments, you rarely take time to just feel satisfied. When triggered, your impatience can push you to work even harder. While you may not make your accomplishments look easy, you do show others that *anything* is attainable with time, patience, and the proper inner resources. Responsibility and duty are key, but are you taking responsibility for your softer side too? Beware of skimping on emotional self-care.

Your Physical Health

As a structure-based sign, you need to establish a consistent health routine. Stay faithful to the rituals that enliven you, particularly your workout routines, diet, and self-care practices. Capricorn rules the bones, so warm baths are especially helpful. Also take extra care of your knees.

Movement that works your balance and helps you bend allows you to carry your authority in a nonthreatening way. It can also prevent you from developing health conditions that result from feeling blocked. Both squats and yoga can support you in these ways. The ruling planet of your sun sign, Saturn, correlates with the skin and teeth too. So dry-brushing your body before you bathe and good oral hygiene go a long way. Saturn goes retrograde yearly, and when he does, it's important for you to reclaim your sovereignty as a path to physical power. But no matter the time of year, stay mindful of your tendency toward rigidity.

♒ AQUARIUS
(JANUARY 20–FEBRUARY 18)
Genius. Revolutionary. Designer.

Symbol: Water Bearer
Element: Air
Ruling Planets: Saturn and Uranus
Mode: Fixed

Your Strengths

Others see you as a little different—and with good reason. Not only do you dance to the beat of your own drum, you encourage the rest of us to make our own music too. Steeped in progressive thinking, you like to take a bird's-eye view of your projects to foster out-of-the-box, big-picture thinking. You're great at capitalizing on diversity, so clearly identify what makes you stand out. Unafraid to ditch convention and break the rules, you aren't here to recklessly throw tradition on its head. You respect what's working and preserve it, while changing what's not. You are a whip-smart, well-ordered genius with a keen eye for detail. Your talent for innovation and your trendsetting sensibility take your work to the next level. With your drive to make a difference, your novel ideas aim to enhance the good of many.

Your Challenges

While your unique perspective is a much-needed gift, you may sometimes struggle to relate to others. If you feel your freedom or individuality is being disrespected, you tend to isolate yourself instead of inviting people into your point of view. Yet it's through relationships that you can truly change the world. Though not always easy for you, developing your emotional acuity supports your artistry, ingenuity, and leadership. You certainly possess the communication skills to connect, Aquarius. It's up to you to break down any barriers that get in your way. Join a group that can make a difference—just not a mainstream one. Focus on finding *your* people.

Your Self-Care

To feel satisfied on this strange and sometimes cumbersome planet, it's key for you to accept the full range of what makes you *you*. Don't ignore those wild flashes of insight or that ping in your chest telling you you're on the right track. Write them down—*all* of them—and give them space to marinate. It's only a matter of time before you connect the realm of possibility to current reality. At times you can be emotionally aloof, so pay attention to your emotions and practice opening up to others. Uranus, the modern ruler of your chart, revolves around the sun in an elliptical pattern that's sideways. It's different. It's opposite. You are similarly oppositional, and this can sometimes feel isolating. Learning to tend to the part of you that feels alone is essential. Uranus goes retrograde annually for approximately five months. During this time, you are asked to integrate what you are learning on your path to liberation. Where in your life can you more fully embrace your authenticity? How can you live more bravely? What can you do to solidify your connection to your emotions? Contemplate the ways you can own your inner strength and rise.

Your Physical Health

Aquarius rules the ankles and calves, which help you remain balanced as you make waves in the world. The ankle contains only three major bones, yet it plays a crucial role in the body by connecting the feet to the lower legs. Similarly, the calves connect the knees to the ankles. To build on this theme of connectivity and apply it more generally to your physical well-being, you are well served by intentionally developing the connection between your mind, body, and emotions. You tend to be more cerebral than emotional and have intellectual and creative break-throughs faster than most. But you live in your head, not your body, and because of this, you miss out on fully integrating your wisdom. Over time, this can lead to feeling ungrounded, edgy, and fried. Perhaps even prone to varicose veins, cold sweats from nervous system overstimula-tion, clumsiness, lack of coordination, swollen ankles, and ankle inju-ries. To offset these tendencies, try slow, mindful movement practices like yin yoga, pilates, strength training, and taking long walks. Strengthen your ankles by doing balancing poses, like yoga's tree pose and ankle circles. Diaphragmatic breathing centers you, strengthening your body's ability to detoxify itself naturally. It also enables you to develop a deeper connection with your emotions—precisely what you need—so you walk your talk and lead the rest of us forward.

♓ PISCES
(FEBRUARY 19–MARCH 20)
Empath. Healer. Poet.

Symbol: Pair of Fish
Element: Water
Ruling Planets: Neptune and Jupiter
Mode: Mutable

Your Strengths

As the last sign of the zodiac, you're born with an innate wisdom that takes the rest of us a lifetime — or several — to accumulate. As a mutable water sign, you easily sense surrounding energy fields, which is why you aren't satisfied with a "normal" life. By regularly transcending your physical body and accessing other energy fields, you can escape your own limitations and experience a wider, multidimensional world. This is like a balm for your overstimulated soul. Ruled by imaginative Neptune and Jupiter, your visions and dreams are potent. You lean toward the arts and spiritual exploration as ways to bring your dreams into reality and process your earthly emotions. Your emotional intelligence and empathy make you a great friend. Between your creative intuition and the depths of your empathy, you have tremendous gifts to share with the world. Give yourself permission to drop the dogmatic baggage and rise. To do so, you have to be grounded — as in, feet-to-earth secure.

Your Challenges

Many traditional religious institutions possess the Piscean undertones of service and sacrifice, but with this conviction comes the idea that being of service is a form of suffering. This is the leftover of thousands of years of misguided religious principles — and this is *not* something for you to harbor within your subconscious. It's imperative that you don't carry that with you in this lifetime. Your sensitivity is your superpower, which means managing it is one of your cosmic lessons, especially when it becomes overwhelming for you. That said, it's essential to be *here*, like on Earth. The mysterious realms of imagination and mysticism tend to sweep you away. Which isn't always a bad thing, so long as it's not your modus operandi 24-7. This includes drinking, escaping through numbing out or sleep, or projecting your pain onto others. Many think you are all soft and no bite. But when you fight, you fight to win, and nobody even realizes you have a weapon. Staying with your emotions helps you navigate the intensity of your feelings IRL.

Your Self-Care

As a mutable water sign, Pisces is prone to the ebb and flow of emotions — and not just your own but the collective consciousness. Sometimes this energy may feel extremely overwhelming and difficult to decipher — which energy is yours and which belongs to someone else? To ground your ideas in the physical plane, you'll need to focus on the union between your spirit, mind, *and* body. Meditation and other mind–body practices remain nonnegotiable for you. It's also important for Pisces to explore the arts to regain emotional equilibrium. Creativity offers you an escape from the overstimulating physical world and allows you to slip into a world of your own making for a break.

Your Physical Health

Pisces rules the feet. So taking care of them is essential. Slather a nourishing cream on your feet (your hands too, while you're at it) to give your toes the spa treatment (try quick-absorbing sea buckthorn and sesame oils) — because your feet are sensitive, just like you. You might even want to make nightly foot massages part of your regular self-care. Speaking of night, sleep is especially important to you. Take good care to give yourself plenty of time to unwind before bed, and pay attention to your dreams. They are embedded with healing messages and perhaps even a direct link to the collective unconscious. You may be prone to foot problems, allergies, addictions, chronic fatigue, sleep disturbances, and maladies that are mysterious or difficult to diagnose. The key to navigating these vulnerabilities is to be grounded in a daily practice that helps you identify your feelings, both emotional and physical, and understand their messages. You are extremely intuitive and have more answers than you know. Speaking of answers, the ruler of your sun sign goes retrograde annually for roughly five months. Use this time to hear the voice of your soul and listen for new dreams emerging.

CHAPTER 7

The Rising Sign

Own Your Awesome

Honoring your desires and learning how to nurture yourself (moon sign) and aligning with your authentic identity and sources of vitality (sun sign) is nowhere near a full description of what those two signs can do for you, yet this already constitutes a radical directive. But what if you took that one step further and turned on your unique brand of awesome?

What if you could sidestep your critical voice and enter into an engaged state of absorption where you're so focused on the task at hand that your inner critic can't distract you?

What if you could build your resilience, enhance your creativity, and boost your energy by cultivating the best, most genuine aspects of who you are?

What if you were so clear on what you needed to feel lit up that you felt fueled by your own agency?

What if you could present yourself to the world with sincerity while simultaneously amplifying what's so very you?

Did you get all of that?

Let's start with the most important point:

You. Are. Awesome.

And you can do all of what I just mentioned, thanks in part to your rising sign.

Your rising sign, also called your ascendant, is the third and final component of your astrological core. Your rising sign represents your physical body, and it animates who you are—your character and how you interact with the world. Please read the sun and moon descriptions of your rising sign too, as they will provide you with more insight regarding your health needs. Additionally, pay extra attention to its ruling planet—it plays a crucial role in helping you "rise" to your greatest potential.

Our Mighty (Yet Often Overlooked) Superpowers

We all have unique ways of being that invigorate, motivate, and light us up—even through the toughest of times. Maybe it's our tenacity, reliability, or poise that helps us stand out the way we do. Maybe it's something else entirely. Regardless, these inborn aspects of our character come through in ways we don't even realize.

When we struggle with health problems, we tend to forget to leverage these innate and unique aspects that make us *us*—these key traits that make us shine. While we may dismiss these attributes in ourselves, they're often the very ones that other people admire in us. They are, after all, the parts of us that function easily and with excellence. Succinctly put, they feed, fuel, and ignite our awesome.

These strengths, this instinctive excellence that runs through each of us, can help us create deeper levels of well-being. Just as the sun represents who we are, and the moon represents our emotional landscape, the rising sign animates how we show up in the world as well as how the world sees us. It tells us about our image and also about the body. It helps to animate our strengths and reveals how to leverage our innate talents on behalf of our well-being. It fuels our purpose in the world. By understanding and integrating the wisdom our rising sign offers us, we can become more embodied and thrive.

While diet culture constantly drums in the message that obtaining a certain size waistline or status symbol is how to become your best, the truth is that your best self is already inside you. It's most evident when you appreciate and amplify what's *already awesome about you*. With practice, over time, you can enhance these parts of yourself even more. Yes, character strengths *can* be developed. They are linked to your inner awesome, and when utilized, they expand your capacity to feel more confident and focus on the positive. They also increase your resilience.

Sound too good to be true? For once it's not.

Understanding Your Rising Sign

Determining your sun sign and your moon sign is relatively straightforward. Your rising sign is trickier. In fact, it's the hardest part of your chart to establish because it's determined by knowing the exact time (down to the minute) and location of your birth. It indicates the zodiac sign that rose on the eastern horizon at the time and place of your birth.

For that reason, the location and time of your birth are essential. Getting as close to the actual minute of your birth is incredibly important, since a rising sign will shift approximately every two hours. There are also thirty degrees within each sign on the tropical zodiac chart. Since the rising sign degree shifts every four minutes, even twins can have slightly different degrees of the same rising sign, or in some rare cases different rising signs altogether.

Your rising sign serves as your first house cusp, a critical angle in your chart. (Knowing your rising becomes more important when you want to work with other techniques.) In the cosmic health framework, it gives you insight into what you're innately excellent at—your awesome—as well as what drives you, and why.

Having a fire sign (Aries, Leo, or Sagittarius) as your rising sign indicates energy, optimism, spontaneity, and enthusiasm as your driving forces. These signs feel best when they're moving fast and have lots of room for creativity. Earth rising signs (Taurus, Capricorn, and Virgo) thrive when they tap into their practical, cautious, and disciplined natures. Relationship and communication skills lead to success for rising air signs (Gemini, Libra, and Aquarius); these signs need verbal interaction, period. Water signs (Pisces, Scorpio, and Cancer) are most energized when using their intuition, empathy, and emotional intelligence.

Knowing your strengths allows you to focus on developing them and achieving goals that will increase both your pleasure and your sense of purpose. It can also provide a deeper sense of what you're meant to do — those goals that are heartfelt and value driven, rather than focused on what you may believe you "should" want.

DON'T KNOW YOUR TIME OF BIRTH?

If you've done everything to find out your time of birth but still don't know it, you can have a qualified astrologer do a chart rectification, which is a highly technical way of determining your birth time. Find an astrologer who's certified through a reputable organization and specializes in chart rectification. Please see the notes at the end of this book for organizations that train people in this astrological specialty.

Cultivating Your Awesome

With or without your rising sign, understanding your character strengths and how they can be used to improve your life is at the core of evidence-based positive psychology.

In 2004, Dr. Martin E. P. Seligman, a University of Pennsylvania professor, and Christopher Peterson, both leaders in the field of positive psychology, went deep into the exploration of human strengths. Looking throughout history and across the globe, they identified six core virtues that all humans share, and the twenty-four character strengths that develop these virtues. While we all possess all of these character strengths, each of us has a unique blend of them, present in varying degrees.

The VIA Character Strengths Survey was created by the VIA Institute on Character, a nonprofit organization led by a distinguished team of psychologists and researchers in positive psychology, the science of thriving. The survey is a free, confidential assessment that's partially based on Seligman's work. Your assessment is specific to you and allows you to determine your core character strengths. Even if you are able to calculate your rising sign, I encourage you to take the survey, which you can do here: viacharacter.org.

A Higher State of Well-Being

Flourishing is viewed as an awareness of, and commitment to, an attuned inner and outer life in which internal needs are met and external demands are negotiated without compromise to physical or mental health.[1]

—CATHERINE P. COOK-COTTONE,
UNIVERSITY AT BUFFALO PROFESSOR

To achieve an even higher level of well-being and truly flourish, we need to live a fulfilling life that aligns with our values and interests as well as our strengths.

Dr. Seligman developed PERMA for this reason. An evidence-based model of well-being, it identifies the five key attributes of flourishing and points the way toward how to develop them. PERMA is an acronym for these building blocks:

P—**Positive Emotions:** Positive emotions lead to higher levels of creativity, resilience, generosity, and success as well as better relationships and physical health.[2] Cultivating gratitude, excitement, and enjoyment increases positive emotions.

E — Engagement: When we leverage our strengths to complete a challenging task, we enter a "flow" state in which we're so engaged that we lose track of everything except the activity at hand. Being in flow is a very healing place to be.

R — Relationships: Nurturing strong, genuine relationships with our parents, siblings, peers, partners, coworkers, and community is essential to our resilience.

M — Meaning: Living for a purpose greater than ourselves gives life meaning. We can find that meaning in spiritual practice(s), social causes, and family, among other things.

A — Accomplishments: Setting our sights on value-driven and heartfelt goals provides the deepest sense of pride and satisfaction once we achieve them.[3]

PERMA isn't exhaustive when it comes to flourishing, but PERMA provides a baseline to understand what it takes to thrive. It will also help you make choices that align with your values and strengths.

To learn more, I recommend reading Seligman's book, *Flourish*.

The Importance of Effort and Practice

One of the most exciting discoveries from Seligman and Peterson's work is that we can practice our strengths and, in doing so, develop them even more. We first need to identify our strengths, and then embrace a growth mindset, which is the belief that we can grow, change, and learn.

The term "growth mindset" was coined by renowned psychologist Carol Dweck, bestselling author of *Mindset: The New Psychology of Success,* to describe students who believed they could get smarter through effort. Individuals with a growth mindset think, *I can learn. I can improve. I can research/study/practice to upgrade my understanding and performance.* The payoff is real: her research clearly demonstrated that students with a growth mindset dedicated more time and attention to their studies and subsequently achieved more.

On the other hand, students with a "fixed mindset" were convinced that their basic qualities, such as their intelligence and talents, were static, so they didn't make additional effort. They thought, *This is all I'll ever be* or *I'm smart already*. Lacking the sustained effort to improve their knowledge and skills, their levels of achievement suffered alongside their self-esteem.

The benefits of the growth mindset make it clear that having character strengths isn't enough; *developing* character strengths is what leads to greater resilience, self-esteem, self-efficacy, and confidence.

As a result, it's important to focus on who you are at your best and practice amplifying it. Look at where you're exceptional and zero in on maximizing it. We're all more likely to succeed when we play to our strengths rather than exclusively trying to remedy our weaknesses.

I learned this firsthand when I left the corporate world to start my own business. Initially, I tried to make it as a yoga teacher. It didn't go well. Moving and adjusting bodies felt burdensome. Sequencing classes didn't excite me. It now seems obvious that yoga wasn't a career path for me, but at the time I wanted to be in the healing arts and "yoga teacher" was the only way I could think of to do that.

Yet I didn't see that incongruity between who I am and the work I was pursuing until I had to withdraw from an intense, advanced yoga-teaching training because of an injury. (In this instance an injury created chaos in my life, disrupting my plans massively and ultimately redirecting my entire existence.) While I was devastated to have to pause my training to heal my shoulder, I used that time to get certified as an Ayurvedic nutritionist. That new training taught me that I thrive in the role of coach. Already aware of my ability to communicate and synthesize complex information, I then applied to a behavior-change health coaching program at Duke Integrative Medicine. That's when my career as an entrepreneur and coach began to gel; as a Libra-rising sign, intimate, one-on-one conversations come naturally to me.

We can all look at where we're exceptional and cultivate those characteristics. Utilizing and amplifying our strengths unlocks our potential to thrive. We become better able to effect change in our lives and develop a greater sense of self-efficacy and self-possession.

When we operate from our strengths and lean into them during difficult times, we can handle the ups and downs of life in constructive ways. Even in the midst of extreme turmoil, we can stay centered and feel better equipped to adapt to stressful situations.

Let's face it, stepping into our power and experiencing true well-being means ditching our attachment to "playing it safe." Instead, we have to put our asses on the line, and to do that we need resilience. Without it, we become susceptible to life circumstances knocking us down and convincing us to give up.

Finding the Fire to Be You

Sometimes we overlook our innate awesome and try to make ourselves fit into an ideal that's not of our own making. When we do so, we lose the fire to cultivate and own our awesome. There's an animated movie titled *Rock Dog* about a father and son who navigate this journey. While the father expresses his fire by fighting to protect his village, the son is drawn to music. This creates a rift in their relationship until...spoiler alert: the son fully owns his awesome and activates his healing magic (his fire) by rocking out to his heart's desire. It's a kid-friendly movie that's fun for adults too. Check it out!

What You're Really Here For

You don't have to be anyone but yourself to be worthy.
—Tarana Burke, founder of the Me Too movement

Many of us fail to take our talents and gifts into account when identifying who we really are. We judge our worth based on our appearance. We define ourselves by the roles we play (parent, friend, partner, boss). We put off pursuing our dreams because we see them as a "one-day" reality instead of a here-and-now probability. Yes, when we disconnect from what drives our soul, we miss out on what's awesome! We all have strengths, and they are waiting to be mastered. As positive psychology research indicates, doing more of what we do well builds self-esteem and a sense of self-mastery, and makes us happier and healthier.

Toward that end, next we'll look at each rising sign in detail.

The Ascendant in Your Natal Chart: Putting It to Work for You

♈ ARIES RISING SIGN
Pioneer. Director. Athlete.

Symbol: Ram
Element: Fire
Ruling Planet: Mars
Mode: Cardinal

With an Aries rising sign, even when you're charging full speed ahead, you inject warmth, optimism, and an unparalleled can-do attitude into just about any situation. People are naturally drawn to your physical presence and sense of adventure. Just be sure you don't leave them in the dust when you take off for your next adventure!

Not everyone is full of boundless energy, and most of us need a little leg up every once in a while. It's important for you to honor your vigor while also understanding that not everyone is as quick on their feet as you are. If there's any zodiac sign that's going to go at it too hard, too fast, it's you. That said, when you don't honor your vitality, you can feel frustrated or even angry. Trust the direction your boundless energy is leading you in—and remember to take a break once in a while—to own your awesome.

Strengths: You are a powerhouse like no other. Others look to you for motivation, for inspiration, and to be catalyzed by your ability to set the world ablaze.

Own-Your-Awesome-Mantra: I trust my vitality.

♉ TAURUS RISING SIGN
Epicurean. Gardener. Aphrodite.

Symbol: Bull
Element: Earth
Ruling Planet: Venus
Mode: Fixed

As a Taurus rising, you aren't short on people who need you. Whether you're cooking a homemade meal or helping friends redecorate their homes, people are drawn to your kind and gentle demeanor. Just be sure you aren't neglecting your own needs in the name of helping others.

More than any other sign, you understand that self-care is the cornerstone of a healthy existence, but it can be hard for you to put away tasks that need finishing and focus on your own needs. Put that hell-bent tenacity to good use and turn off the phone, draw a bubble bath, and indulge in a lush novel.

Once you've restored yourself, get back to work ASAP. As a Taurus rising, there isn't an indulgence you wouldn't like to dip your toes into, and after caring for others all day, you definitely deserve it. For extra motivation, enlist your senses with a candle burning on your desk or a few squares of dark chocolate waiting as your reward.

Strengths: You have a genuine warmth and exude honesty. Others feel safe in your presence, allowing you to bond easily and develop sincere relationships.

Own-Your-Awesome-Mantra: I trust my senses.

♊ GEMINI RISING SIGN
Networker. Teacher. Writer.

Symbol: Twins
Element: Air
Ruling Planet: Mercury
Mode: Mutable

With abundant social graces, a Gemini rising can talk to just about anyone. Versatile, creative, and never short on words, you bring a quicksilver energy to any situation or person interesting enough to hold your attention. This tendency to flit from idea to idea may appear flighty, but in truth it's partly your insatiable curiosity that fuels your awe-inspiring mind.

Whatever the reasons, you're happiest when hopscotching between multiple realms of ideas and people — both Gemini specialties. You like to take an idea from one place and sprinkle it into an unlikely situation. You're also keen to mix, match, and experiment with modes of communication in order to invent something totally new.

This tendency to move between people and projects satiates your creative instinct; just be sure your curiosity isn't mistaken for disingenuity. You're most powerful when you combine that curious mind with your opposite sign, Sagittarius, which has a knack for finding the best in others. You don't need to know *everything* about everyone; sometimes it's best to see what they can become.

Strengths: Aside from being a natural networker, your intellect leads the way as you bridge ideas in ways previously unthought of.

Own-Your-Awesome-Mantra: I trust my curiosity.

♋ CANCER RISING SIGN
Empress. Breadwinner. Nurturer.

Symbol: Crab
Element: Water
Ruling Planet: Moon
Mode: Cardinal

With a Cancer rising sign, you require a strong foundation. This means you can come off as a homebody who likes to play her cards close to the vest. It's not that you're incapable of dreaming big or taking bold leaps; you just prefer to build a solid base first.

You're not just stellar at building a nest egg for the future; you excel at nesting, period. Your home is almost always rich with warm colors and soft textures. Even if you don't consider yourself to be a "homemaker" in the traditional sense, your loved ones likely see you as the embodiment of a safe place where they can rest, reflect, and heal.

Your emotions tend to be all-encompassing, so you aren't into sharing them with just anyone. You have to totally trust someone before you'll open up (again with that sense of security). There's nothing wrong with that, as long as you're still willing to grow through your relationships. You don't always have to be the one doing the protecting—allow others to care for you too.

> *Strengths:* Your bones are made of wisdom. While you have a level of emotional intelligence that's off the charts, you're certainly not soft all of the time. You blend devotion and grit seamlessly.

> *Own-Your-Awesome-Mantra:* I trust my tenacity.

♌ LEO RISING SIGN
Sovereign. Motivator. Leader.

Symbol: Lion
Element: Fire

Ruling Planet: Sun
Mode: Fixed

With a Leo rising sign, there's no spotlight you won't naturally drift toward. Not only are you comfortable with all eyes in your direction, you require it, and with good reason—people see you as a leader.

Your magnetism and natural charm make it easy for you to collect followers anywhere you go. People tend to reach for your warmth as a way to build up their own confidence. And let's face it, you don't mind the ego stroke either. As you grow into your own confidence, it's important to remember to lead with integrity and morality. Also, take a cue from your opposite sign, Aquarius, by learning to serve the collective good, first and foremost.

One way you can have a far-reaching impact is by putting your fun-loving nature to good use. You innately understand and respect the all-important roles of fun and freedom. You have the power to show the rest of the world that even the toughest climb to the top can be made more bearable with a lighthearted attitude.

Strengths: You are here to set the world ablaze. Full of vitality and strength, you are naturally optimistic. This serves your ability to lead with courage and power.

Own-Your-Awesome-Mantra: I trust in my ability to lead.

♍ VIRGO RISING SIGN
Mentor. Engineer. Editor.

Symbol: Virgin
Element: Earth
Ruling Planet: Mercury
Mode: Mutable

As a Virgo rising, you aren't just organized; your budget is color-coded, and the clothes in your closet are steam pressed and arranged by season.

Some people may see you as nitpicky, but that's not really the case. In truth, you can't stand excess. Everything has a purpose—you just have to uncover it.

As the "protector of purity," you prefer to streamline *everything*, especially your day-to-day operations. You have a knack for identifying and cutting away anything that won't propel you toward your goals. What's more, people respect you for it.

In true Virgo fashion, you often find yourself drawn to service-oriented careers and projects. Even if you aren't working in a traditional "service" industry, you may be signing up for volunteer committees or finding ways to help people set up their spreadsheets and streamline their calendars. Just be sure not to let the daily grind get in the way of thinking of the bigger picture.

> *Strengths:* Your attention to detail, work ethic, and sense of service make you incredibly valuable—not just to those in your inner circle but all you serve with your purpose.

> *Own-Your-Awesome-Mantra:* I trust my devotion to service.

♎ LIBRA RISING SIGN
Artist. Advocate. Liberator.

Symbol: Scales
Element: Air
Ruling Planet: Venus
Mode: Cardinal

If there's anyone who looks like they've got it all together, it's a Libra rising. From your killer wardrobe to your epic art collection, you know what it means to honor the sophistication of the human spirit.

Not only can you find soul essence in canvases and couture, you're also excellent at bringing out the best in your fellow humans. Relationships are your domain, and people of all walks of life tend to flock to you. You make them feel comfortable in their own skin. It's healing through radical acceptance.

For your rising sign in particular, you'll need to pay special attention to the way you expend your energy. Balance is key, and your many friends, family, and flyby acquaintances will try to take up every bit of your free time—if you let them. You'll need to find equilibrium between the internal and external, as well as between your finely honed social graces and your necessarily firm boundaries, to keep you healthy and happy for the long run.

Strengths: Your diplomatic nature can see both sides of any coin, and your compassion is a guiding force. You are judicious by nature, and abide by a commitment to peace.

Own-Your-Awesome-Mantra: I trust my judicious nature.

♏ SCORPIO RISING SIGN
Sorceress. Therapist. Investigator.

Symbol: Scorpion
Element: Water
Ruling Planets: Pluto and Mars
Mode: Fixed

With Scorpio as your rising sign, there's no stone unturned, no closet unexplored. It's not that you're nosy—quite the contrary. You only seek confirmation of what you already know deep within.

This inner knowing is so innate that it seeps into your personality. To those around you, you come across as wise beyond your years, almost as if this isn't your first go-round in human form. And even though you give off the vibe that you know something others don't, you're still keenly observant. There's nothing that gets by you. You take note of even the most inconsequential details and store them in your massive internal database for later use.

Even with your firm grasp of the human psyche, you can come across as guarded. It's not that you don't enjoy other people; it's just that your watery nature tends to absorb *everything*. You feel deeply, and while that is one of your strengths, it can also breed fear. Allow yourself to be imperfect, let things go, and experience life instead of keeping everything under wraps.

Strengths: There's no situation that's too dark, too scary, or beyond your ability to handle. While you may doubt this, and sometimes crumble in the face of fire, give yourself a break. You are stronger than you think!

Own-Your-Awesome-Mantra: I trust my inner knowing.

↗ SAGITTARIUS RISING SIGN
Bon Vivant. Teacher. Truth Seeker.

Symbol: Archer
Element: Fire
Ruling Planet: Jupiter
Mode: Mutable

As a Sagittarius rising sign, your zest for life is a highlight of your outward personality. People love to be around you—and why wouldn't they? Not only do you come off as fun loving and jovial, but also you're not afraid to wax philosophical about the deeper truths of our existence.

And all this talk about big-picture ideas didn't come for free, Sag. You've gone out and explored the world for yourself—whether through tomes or train rides. That's why people inherently trust your worldview. On some level, they understand that you practice what you preach, so they're willing to trust you with the task of injecting them with a fresh perspective.

Even in your healthiest relationships, you're pretty tough to pin down. Freedom is your driving force, you know how to expand, and no one can hold you back. Stay honest, work hard, and build a life you love around that innate urge for freedom and adventure.

Strengths: Your jovial nature finds the silver lining, making you not just a natural optimist but someone who can leverage what's going right with ease and grace. While those around you are fixated on the flaw, you quickly find the solution.

Own Your Awesome Mantra: I trust my ability to discern the truth.

♑ CAPRICORN RISING SIGN
Expert. Strategist. Executive.

Symbol: Sea Goat
Element: Earth
Ruling Planet: Saturn
Mode: Cardinal

With a Capricorn rising, it's best if everyone just gets out of your way while you handle it all. At least, that's the way people tend to perceive you like you're a leader who knows what you're doing.

You're dedicated and devoted, and you know that it's only a matter of time until you can add "CEO" to your email signature. Some people may see this attitude of inevitable success as arrogant, but that's only because you haven't clued them in to just how many behind-the-scenes hours you're really putting in, Cap.

You prefer order over discord, structure over winging it. Because of this, others may see you as a bit of a fun slayer. It's not that you don't enjoy a good time...once you're there. Your disciplined nature knows how to get it done, making it hard to pull you away from your desk, especially when you're passionate about your projects. Pencil in a night out once in a while, and let yourself unwind. Let's face it: your success is likely.

Strengths: Tenacity is your middle name. Once you know what you want, you don't give up or back down. This makes you an asset not just professionally but also in your family and community.

Own-Your-Awesome-Mantra: I trust my grit.

♒ AQUARIUS RISING SIGN
Genius. Revolutionary. Designer.

Symbol: Water Bearer
Element: Air
Ruling Planets: Saturn and Uranus
Mode: Fixed

As an Aquarius rising, some think you march to the beat of your own drum. In reality, you've ditched the drum altogether and are rock and rolling it out with an electronic soundboard—one that you built with spare parts, of course. You're an inventor, innovator, and icon. And sometimes people just aren't sure what to do with you.

Despite their initial tentativeness, people eventually flock to you. They sense that there's truth at the core of your wild ideas, and that you just may be the Next Big Thing. Even if people aren't interested in riding on your coattails, they understand there's something unique about the way you perceive the world. And they want to know more about it—and you.

While you may be seen as a visionary, you're also excellent at making connections between seemingly dissimilar ideas, people, and places. It's easy for you to see how all the dots connect to make the world a better place. You're just waiting for everyone else to get on board.

Strengths: You are here to show people what's possible. You have always been and probably always will be ahead of the curve. You don't settle for mediocrity; instead, you have your sights set on how to make things better.

Own-Your-Awesome-Mantra: I trust my ingenuity.

♓ PISCES RISING SIGN

Empath. Healer. Poet.

Symbol: Pair of Fish
Element: Water
Ruling Planets: Neptune and Jupiter
Mode: Mutable

With your rising sign in ethereal Pisces, you seem to know everything, but not in the traditional, masculine sense. Your knowledge comes from somewhere beyond this place—a spiritual gift received, not attained.

You're a sensitive soul who's quick to feel overwhelmed, but that's not necessarily a bad thing. Because you feel so deeply, you have empathy like no other, are extremely artistic, and can always count on your intuition to know best. You're at your best when you can stay true to your spiritual practices. Or when you gather with a small group of trusted friends, preferably somewhere healing, like the shoreline of a gently lapping ocean.

You feel at home in healing places because you, too, are a natural healer. Others sense this about you, so don't be surprised if anyone and everyone shows up to dump their energetic baggage on you. While you prefer to go with the flow, it's best if you learn to set some firm boundaries when it comes to your energy. A healer is no good to anyone if she can't care for herself.

Strengths: You know, in your body, exactly what's lying beneath the surface for others. You immediately pick up on unspoken nuances. Because of this, your artistic, intuitive, and healing capacities are enviable.

Own-Your-Awesome-Mantra: I trust my intuition.

Ritual: Own Your Awesome

Now that you have learned more about yourself through the lens of your core astrology and character strengths, take a moment to digest your discoveries. You can do this at your altar if you'd like, though it's not necessary for this ritual.

Here are some questions for you to consider.

What is my sun sign?

What is my moon sign?

What is my rising sign?

What is the ruling planet of my rising sign? How do I relate to this planet?

What are my top-five signature strengths? Of these strengths, which do I feel most called to master at this moment of my life?

What element is associated with each sign?

Sun:

Moon:

Rising:

What mode is associated with each sign?

Sun:

Moon:

Rising:

Of these three signs, which do I feel I relate to most and why?

How can I best leverage the strengths associated with my core astrology?

Based on the combination of my sun, moon, rising sign, and character strength, what's my unique blend of awesome?

Make a list of your superpowers. How are you uniquely awesome? Doing this might feel awkward at first, especially if you aren't used to celebrating yourself. Be patient, and keep going.

Once your list is complete, consider a struggle you are facing. Maybe it's a health challenge, or a challenge with self-confidence. Like so many, perhaps, you are struggling with a career issue or a relationship dynamic. The goal is to identify one area where you are currently seeking improvement.

Once you've identified an area of life that you want to improve, look at your superpowers again. How can you apply your unique brand of awesome to this issue? What strength, skill, natural talent, or ability can you develop and use even more? Using your strengths and applying them to your problems will help you grow, supporting you to create the lasting change you seek.

Now, commit. Craft an affirmation or a mantra that positively reinforces your innate talent, and your ability to make the desired change. Then, say it out loud and meditate on it. See yourself fully realizing your potential and owning your awesome. Most important, though, visualize yourself actively using your strengths in the context of the problem you want to solve. See the ways you can, and will, apply your strengths to triumph.

Once you feel resolute, thank yourself. Give yourself love, gratitude, and appreciation for all the ways you are already *awesome*!

Now that you have your astrological core — your moon, sun, and rising signs — you're ready to move into part IV, where we'll go deeper into your chart and how it supports your cosmic health.

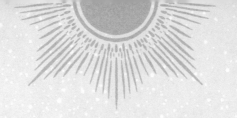

Part IV

WATER

Harnessing Planetary Wisdom in Your Life

Freedom is just chaos with better lighting.
—Alan Dean Foster, from *To the Vanishing Point*

CHAPTER 8

Mercury

Can You Really Have What You Want?

H ow long are you going to waste time here in idle luxury?" Hermes, the Greek messenger god, asked in his most severe voice. "The ruler of heaven himself has sent me to you. He bids you depart and seek the kingdom which is your destiny."[1]

Hermes was speaking to Aeneas, but he could just as easily have been speaking to you, me—or any of us, really.

Have you ever felt a calling so deep it seemed to come from a divine source? Have you ever felt so inspired to pursue something that it was like a spiritual mandate? That calling may be a new career, motherhood, a creative project, or an epic trip—and often, several of those, and more, over the course of a lifetime.

While we may not be gods or goddesses in a mythological sense, we *do* have superpowers. Once we're willing, as we've seen, we *can* own our awesome. That often means seeking our own "kingdom" and realizing our own "destiny."

Yet so often we hesitate and procrastinate; we put it off for another month, another season, another year. Why do we do this?

While we may "idle in luxury" to avoid hard work, even when our bigger hopes and dreams don't require significant sacrifice, a lot of us tend to linger and stall.

In this chapter, we'll explore this tendency and how it relates to mindset, as well as the all-important role of the "messenger planet," Mercury, in getting what we most desire. Last but not least, we'll look at how your natal Mercury placement can help you proactively move toward what you truly want.

However, before we do, I want to share a few thoughts on how systemic oppression affects the seeking of our kingdom and the realizing of our destiny.

On Mindset and Privilege

As we delve into the topic of mindset, it's important to acknowledge the very real external influences stemming from racism, and other biases, that limit our power to create change and to realize our individual destinies.

Systemic injustices and oppression are impediments to cosmic health. Designed to keep us unwell, they damage the well-being of the collective and gravely affect the individual health of Black, Brown, and Indigenous populations, especially for those who identify as women, are a part of the LGBTQ community, suffer with mobility impairment, or lack economic agency. We absolutely must take individual and collective *action* to disrupt systems of oppression so we can realize our collective destiny.

While this is a chapter on mindset, I am not suggesting we can *think* our way out of oppression, widespread inequality, or the many injustices plaguing society. In this chapter, however, we focus on the personal planet Mercury, who represents our ability to reason, which in the cosmic health framework translates as optimizing our mindset to support, even boost, our individual well-being.

Mindset is a tool of resilience, which allows us to face life exactly as it is, however hard it may be, and stay committed to the path of rising, on behalf of both our individual and our collective health. While mind-set cannot negate the historical and present-day impact of racism, it, like Mercury, can help each of us to adjust our beliefs so they support us in pursuit of our collective liberation. This allows us to confront the very real societal limitations on freedom with even more resilience.

Opening Up to Abundance

Early in my coaching career I discovered an interesting underlying theme among my clients. Many wanted to reach a milestone in their lives, yet they were afraid that obtaining their goal would translate into heartbreak or loss in some other part of their lives. Outwardly, these women were accomplished, confident, and impressive. Yet many of them secretly believed that as soon as they'd "used up" their maximum allow-ance of abundance, bad stuff would begin to happen.

This belief can play out in any number of ways. For Emma, a Dutch woman who lived in Amsterdam, it translated into resistance around addressing her emotional eating. As a mental health professional, she'd long used nighttime snacking as a way to relax and unwind from her fulfilling but draining work. Yet over the years, that habit had become an unhealthy way of avoiding her feelings. It had also contributed to a deep discomfort with her own body. Emma felt increasingly powerless to stop her binge eating, and that perceived loss of control had slowly but surely eroded her self-esteem.

As we worked together, we discovered additional resistance around addressing her emotional eating. Since grade school, Emma had inter-nalized the idea that the "it" girls, all of whom had been thin and seem-ingly perfect, had seemed to forsake their intelligence and individuality in order to be slim. Rather than follow suit, she'd opted to be gutsy, artsy, and interesting. That choice had served her well, yet, unconsciously, it also had become her permission slip to use candy to avoid processing her feelings.

Emma began to explore a new relationship with her emotions and food. She realized that candy was a cheap substitute for joy and that she could make lifestyle changes without forsaking pleasure. By practicing feeling her feelings without using emotional eating to numb out, she experienced a noticeable shift in her energy. Her confidence increased as she found more bravery within.

So often we build mental blocks around what we're allowed to have—financial and professional success, but not true love; health, but not pleasure; a life partner, but not our ideal lifestyle. These limiting beliefs hold us back, convincing us that we're obligated to forsake at least one of our dreams or desires in order to have another.

While we may have to make various changes at different times in order to get what we desire, sacrificing ourselves, our health, and our dreams does *not* have to be part of the process. Once we release these either-or limiting beliefs around how much good we're "allowed" to have, we find that the changes we do have to make, while awkward at first, are more possible than we previously assumed. While the outcome is never a guarantee, there's so much joy in trying.

Breaking Through Our Upper Limit

Gay Hendricks, the author of *The Big Leap*, calls the limitations we place on how good our lives can be our "upper limit." That upper limit is the ceiling we all have around how good we can let ourselves feel. Once we get to that point, we find a way to sabotage even our best efforts and most prized achievements, too afraid of loss and pain to risk venturing further. This speaks to why we assume we must sacrifice at least one part of ourselves and our dreams to get another—unconsciously, we're committed to our limits.

I've experienced this incongruence at different times and in different ways in my own life. After returning from my world travels and moving to New York City, my love life was stronger than ever, yet I felt increasingly hopeless about pursuing my career. For a while I internalized the idea that I could have a great relationship *or* a great career, but not both.

Eventually I noticed an even deeper, more limiting belief that I later discovered many of my clients also harbor — that by holding ourselves back in some way, we may be able to "control" the amount of suffering we experience. This, of course, is a profoundly false belief. The truth is, we all experience suffering and loss in life. By spending our lives trying to limit these negative emotions, we often increase our disappointment and despair. Once I realized that I *could* have a partnership and a career I love — that the upper limit I'd faced previously was one I'd created myself — I also realized I didn't need to try to "control" my suffering.

Turning Fear and Resistance into Treasure

Looking back, I can see that my career transition, while major, was also sort of simple — once I'd shifted my mindset and wholeheartedly pursued my desires. Some big changes are like that, and some are not. About ten years later, I found myself at a crossroads that didn't feel so easy.

It began one day as I sat before my gynecologist and she uttered "osteoporosis." Hearing that word, I froze in shock and horror.

Osteoporosis, a disease common among older women, occurs when bones become so brittle, they can fracture from simple movement, like bending forward. While I knew that osteoporosis was a risk after my hysterectomy, I'd gone to great lengths over the years to prevent the disease — changing my diet, supplementing with bioequivalent estrogen and vitamins, working out, practicing yoga, and seeing specialty doctors. But none of that could make up for not having actual ovaries.

Although I was only in my thirties, my bones were growing increasingly brittle. That diagnosis was a huge blow to my confidence, and it propelled me into an existential crisis. For months I battled massive waves of fear, anxiety, grief, and anger that felt like an emotional flood

I couldn't escape. Knowing that my health would require a tremendous amount of my energy and attention from that point forward, I agonized over whether or not to pursue adoption. It was a grueling choice.

Unlike with my business, this time I wouldn't get what I wanted — not even close. It's a reality that many people with chronic illnesses face. Taking on parenting didn't feel like the right choice for my body. It was a *very* tough decision but ultimately the one I needed to make.

Yet even without a chronic disease, life eventually serves up circumstances that are beyond our control. When that happens, we have a critical choice to make around the kind of story we tell ourselves and the mindset we adopt.

Reframing Our Narratives

Was I existentially cursed, doomed to be dragged down by my physical body, or just being forced to write a new story that didn't yet feel easy, natural, or even right? Questions like that often haunt us in hard times, and for months I, too, struggled to digest my new reality and what it meant for me, my life, and my future.

While we can't always control outcomes, we can control how resilient we're willing to become in the face of challenge and crisis. Knowing this, I eventually shifted my focus to writing the next chapter of my life. Now that motherhood was off the table, what did I want? I could choose either to grieve and rage endlessly or to live the crap out of the good times and enjoy every drop of each day I have.

I won't lie — sometimes that's really hard to do, especially in the face of deep heartbreak and grief, both of which overwhelmed me as I grappled with the reality that I'd never be a mother. Yet even then, I, and all of us, have that essential choice to make: are we going to commit to suffering or to joy, hope, and the abundance that comes from setting a new upper limit?

The Power of Mindset

You know that chart you have to read when you go the eye doctor, the one with a big letter at the top and a row of the tiniest letters at the bottom? From a mindset perspective, that chart tells your brain that you're about to be unable to see, that failure is inevitable and also right around the corner.

Dr. Ellen Langer, a brilliant researcher and psychology professor at Harvard University, wondered what would happen if that same chart was turned upside down. In other words, if the brain immediately got the message that it was about to see very well, and succeed on the vision test, would the actual test results change?

If this sounds unlikely, think about it: when you feel prepared and primed to succeed, do you generally perform better or worse than when failure feels likely, if not inevitable? Have you ever amazed yourself after committing to a goal and achieved feats that previously seemed unimaginable?

As Dr. Langer had foreseen, once the vision test chart was reversed—with the tiniest letters at the top and the largest letter at the bottom—study participants were able to see small letters that they previously hadn't been able to.

The interesting thing about this experiment, and others like it, is that without these kinds of studies we're generally not inclined to question what we think we know or have been told is "reality" or "truth." We take a vision test, get results, and accept them as a straightforward report on the state of our vision. As Langer explains, "We're unaware of when we're mindless...when we're not there, we're not there to know we're not there."[2]

When we're mindless, we accept assumptions and past experiences as "facts" or "truth" rather than considering the current context and circumstances from a fresh perspective. In the case of the eye exam experiment, it means assuming that eye test results are universally valid.

This mindless reliance on past experience and other limiting beliefs is also what keeps us stuck at our upper limit around how much health, joy, success, and/or love we feel we're "allowed" to experience. If we haven't been physically fit before, we believe we never will be. If our intimate relationships have always ended in betrayal and heartache, we believe that, as the song says, "love hurts," and so on.

These are all forms of learned mindlessness, which shows us only what we believe and what we've experienced and blinds us to what's actually possible.

Changing How and What We Think

In Dr. Langer's exploration of what she calls "the psychology of possibility," she also investigated the power of subtle changes in thinking. In her famous 1979 Counterclockwise Study, Dr. Langer brought two groups of elderly men to spend a week at a secluded monastery that was outfitted as if it were 1959. The experimental group was encouraged to act as if they were truly living in 1959, while the control group was encouraged to simply reminisce.

Compared to the control group, the experimental group showed significant improvements in their physical health, including reduced arthritic symptoms, improved vision, higher intelligence test performance, and positive changes to posture and weight. When asked to compare photos of the study participants from the beginning and end of the week, objective observers noted that the experimental group looked noticeably younger after the study. A simple shift in mindset helped this group act, look, and feel younger—with health benchmarks that reflected a more youthful state.[3]

The results were groundbreaking, putting mind–body health at the forefront at a time when it was hardly being discussed. Since then, further studies have supported the idea that mindset and physical health are inextricably linked. Here are just some of them:

- Dr. Langer demonstrated that subjects who were primed to consider themselves air force pilots performed better on an eyesight test after a flight simulation, compared to those who were told to simply pretend to fly a plane.[4]

- A 2016 study showed the blood-glucose levels of people with type 2 diabetes would spike and dip based on perceived time, rather than actual time. The biochemistry of the study participants literally changed in coordination with participants' expectations.[5]

- Another of Dr. Langer's ongoing studies consistently found that individuals who were encouraged to act as if they had a cold, while watching videos of people with cold and flu symptoms, later developed actual symptoms and higher levels of the IgA antibody, which suggests the body was preparing to fight an infection. Those in the control group, who watched only videos without any mindset priming, did not experience these symptoms or an elevated immune response.[6]

With a subtle change in mindset, we can transform our health, advance our abilities, and surpass previous physiological limits. Wow! With this understanding of the power of mindset as a baseline, imagine how else we can improve our health and our lives!

The beautiful truth is, we really *don't* know what we're capable of achieving, and getting started is as simple as nudging ourselves in the right direction. Now, and as often as possible, focus on *doing* something to support your desired mindset shift. Whether that means telling a trusted confidante how you feel, accepting your imperfections, or taking a break to recover emotionally, each small step forward supports the next step. Soon enough, you'll be further along than you could have imagined at the outset.

Using Self-Expression to Shift Mindset

Mindset consists of the attitudes and mental framing we use to filter and interpret information. Our self-expression—how we communicate—is how we broadcast our ideas and beliefs to ourselves and others.

We touched briefly on the importance of self-expression for

emotional health in chapter 5. Indeed, bottling up thoughts and feelings can wreak havoc on our health. Dr. James W. Pennebaker, the social psychologist who has explored the health benefits of expressing yourself through journaling, has paved the way for further exploration into how self-expression influences well-being. As it turns out, communication— verbal and nonverbal—supports us in both physical healing and emotional resilience. Just by expressing ourselves, we support powerful mindset shifts that can improve our health and happiness.

Consider some of these ways of using self-expression to move toward a more empowering mindset:

Journaling: In a 1985 study conducted by Pennebaker and a colleague, college students were asked to write for fifteen minutes per day for four consecutive days about the most traumatic or upsetting event of their entire lives. Compared to the control group, which was asked to write about superficial topics, the experimental group became sick less often and made fewer subsequent visits to the campus health center.[7]

Art and Music: Playing or listening to music and creating art or engaging it as a participant brings you into a deeper connection with the present moment, helping you to become more mindful. As Ellen Langer's research has proven, elevating mindfulness positively impacts well-being through multiple mind-body measures, notably by increasing memory, lowering anxiety, and shifting mood.

What are your go-to modes of self-expression? What resonates with you? We tend to see these activities as an indulgence or a casual hobby. In fact, the ways we engage with self-expression either enable or limit these avenues of release, which in turn affects our health.

As we dive into these all-important areas of mindset and self-expression, we'll look next at Mercury, which you can think of as your cosmic ally who knows exactly how to master them in service of your most vibrant health and happiness.

ADDITIONAL STEPS TOWARD TRANSFORMING YOUR MINDSET

In addition to self-expression, these actions can help you shift your mindset:

1. **Act as if.** Go beyond pretending or musing. Instead, conduct yourself as if you have already achieved your desired outcome(s): an absence of pain, a deeply loving relationship. Consider yourself already living the outcome(s) you desire.

2. **Change your environment.** Match your surroundings with your desired mindset. This can be as simple as clearing out clutter, rearranging a room, or painting one wall an accent color that soothes, inspires, or excites you. It can also mean taking a walk on your favorite trail more often or spending more time with people who lift you up rather than deplete you.

3. **Consider your language.** The words we use are powerful. They influence our perception of our current reality as well as our future expectations.

Mercury, Messenger Planet

As you integrate these new ways of shifting your mindset, you can also look to your natal Mercury placement to guide you.

Mercury, along with Venus and Mars, which we'll explore in the next chapters, are referred to as the "personal" planets. Alongside our natal moon, sun, and rising signs, these three planets combined influence how we think, love, act, and react.

Mercury animates our perception and, because of this, also our mindset. It is the cosmic gatherer of all information and, as the messenger, also the storyteller.

The placement of Mercury in your natal chart reveals the way you communicate with others and how you interact with your environment intellectually and socially. The sign and house placement of your natal Mercury describes the way you focus your mind, what stimulates you to learn, and what you like to learn about.

No big deal, right?

Traveling very close to the sun, Mercury not only influences you in critical ways, it's also a fast-moving planet, completing its orbit around the sun (in its sidereal cycle) in just eighty-eight days. Because Mercury is so close to the sun (in the synodic cycle), it's extremely common to have Mercury in the same sign as your sun sign. If your Mercury sign is different from your sun sign, it's either in the sign ahead of or behind your sun sign.

Using Mercury as your guide, you can learn how to tell your stories in ways that don't make you the victim. Instead, you can see your story as a source of empowerment, and in so doing, shift your mindset to realize your desires.

Emma, the client I mentioned at the beginning of this chapter, with her natal Mercury in Virgo, was both self-critical and very practical. To change her relationship with nighttime snacking, she needed to acknowledge the suffering her inner critic caused her. Not an easy task for anyone, but especially those with Mercury in Virgo. Yet, by becoming more aware of her emotions and needs, she was able to become more compassionate and make meaningful changes.

This required her to become more tolerant of challenging emotions. Once she did, she replaced an old belief that told her feeling good in her body meant being vapid. In doing so, she grew her resilience and began to forge a new relationship with food, pleasure, and feeling good in her body.

Mercury in Your Natal Chart: Putting It to Work for You

Mercury rules the signs of Gemini and Virgo. As the planet that governs analytical thought, learning, and the mind, Mercury's placement in your natal chart offers insight into your mindset and communication style.

Once you know where Mercury falls in your natal chart, look at the following descriptions to discover what your Mercury sign means for you. I have separated each natal Mercury placement into the associated sun signs, plus, in addition to a description, I have included an affirmation for each.

Mercury in Aries ♈

If Mercury traveled in the sign of Aries (cardinal fire) at the time of your birth, you have a Pisces, Aries, or Taurus sun sign.

With quick-witted Mercury in the first sign of the zodiac, you love speed and have the ability to make decisions quickly. You have the capacity to motivate and inspire others.

If you are a Pisces sun sign with Mercury in Aries, you have astute emotional intelligence and the capacity to be assertive too. You know your feelings and can leverage them toward self-understanding and the understanding of others.

> *Your affirmation:* I have the capacity to understand and antici-pate the needs of others and make critical decisions with clarity, decisively. I value my ability to be assertive. I speak with integrity without threatening the integrity of others.

If you are an Aries sun sign with Mercury in Aries, look out, world. You are aware of what you want and not afraid to ask for it. You can com-municate in a bold and blunt way, giving clear direction, yet sometimes you can come off as abrupt. Learning how to slow down is essential.

Your affirmation: I know what I want, and I am confident asking for what I need. I understand that just because it might not show up right away, it doesn't mean it's not coming. I cultivate patience and stay faithful to my dreams.

If you are a Taurus sun sign with Mercury in Aries, life can at times feel jolting, like you have one foot on the gas and the other on the brake. Your grounded disposition means you shy away from risk, but Mercury in Aries means you might engage in risk more than you realize.

Your affirmation: I leverage my steadfast, committed nature while understanding that change is the only constant in life. I conjure the life I wish to live as I allow my heart to heal from past pain and emotional tumult. It's safe for me to desire all that I want.

Mercury in Taurus ♉

If Mercury traveled in the sign of Taurus (fixed earth) at the time of your birth, you have an Aries, Taurus, or Gemini sun sign.

Mercury in Taurus brings grounded vibes, supporting you to nurture further, in addition to nourishing and cultivating, your ideas.

If you are an Aries sun sign with Mercury in Taurus, your sun sign is fiery, while Mercury roots you in steadfast, earth-bound Taurus. Even though you want what you want, like, yesterday, you also possess an incredible sense of patience and commitment.

Your affirmation: Even though I want what I want now, if not sooner, I am capable of staying the course that conjuring my highest destiny and desires requires. I am steadfast and consistent. What I want, wants me.

If you are a Taurus sun sign with Mercury in Taurus, you have fixed earth energy, meaning you favor routine over adventure, yet you have an elevated sense of taste and the capacity to savor the good in life.

Your affirmation: I know that my physical health is my most important asset, and I take care of my body accordingly. I eat for nourishment, sleep for rejuvenation, move for pleasure, and meditate for alignment. I live in sync with the rhythms that guide my life. I do not rush, and that's okay.

If you are a Gemini sun sign with Mercury in Taurus, your quick-witted nature answers to Mercury in one of its most grounded signs. This combination means that in spite of your Gemini sun sign, you favor routine.

Your affirmation: Freedom means having a quiet mind and a fulfilled heart. Therefore, I accept that in this moment I have everything I need to express the full realization of my life. Knowing that my routine and habits make me who I am, I choose them wisely, surrendering that which I no longer need.

Mercury in Gemini ♊

If Mercury traveled in the sign of Gemini (mutable air) at the time of your birth, you have a Taurus, Gemini, or Cancer sun sign.

Since Mercury rules Gemini, Mercury can do his job exceptionally well in this sign. Quick-witted communication and linguistic capacities are the hallmark of anyone with Mercury in this sign.

If you are a Taurus sun sign with Mercury in Gemini, know that Mercury amplifies one of Taurus's hallmark traits: a beautiful voice. When you speak, people listen. Own your point of view, ask for what you need, and do not be afraid to give direction.

Your affirmation: I am grounded and stable, yet I also allow my intelligence to guide me. My quicksilver mind maneuvers problem-solving with practicality and ingenuity.

If you are a Gemini sun sign with Mercury in Gemini, well then, hello there, Gemini! With Mercury in his home and as the ruler of your sun, your lightning-fast intellect remains one of your greatest attributes. Think, write, promote. Use your incredible capacity to teach to your advantage.

> *Your affirmation:* My intellect and verbal capacity are my core strengths. I leverage my discernment, trust my intuition, and listen deeply. My actions are guided by my awareness and a keen sense of perception. When the going gets tough, I recommit to my desires.

If you are a Cancer sun sign with Mercury in Gemini, your Cancer sun sign cherishes memories, loved ones, and nourishment while your Mercury in Gemini keeps you on the go. This can, at times, feel a wee bit conflicting, but here's the deal: your emotional intelligence is off the chain, and you can always find the words to express yourself.

> *Your affirmation:* My emotional intelligence guides my thoughts, words, and actions. I nourish myself through the actualization of my desires. Even when I am discouraged, I stay the course of my desires.

Mercury in Cancer ♋

If Mercury traveled in the sign of Cancer (cardinal water) at the time of your birth, you have a Gemini, Cancer, or Leo sun sign.

Mercury in Cancer amplifies your ability to listen to others and to communicate in a caring manner; use these skills to your advantage. But take time to truly hear before you react.

If you are a Gemini sun sign with Mercury in Cancer, you have the qualities of a quick-witted Gemini, yet you're not even the least bit superficial. You feel deeply, and when you make a commitment to someone or something, you keep it.

> *Your affirmation:* When I make a commitment, I keep it, therefore I think things through before saying yes, and I say yes to

what I really want. I am an excellent listener, and I use this skill to my advantage, always.

If you are a Cancer sun sign with Mercury in Cancer, you have congruence between body and mind. Your gift? Your ability to listen with discernment. Your challenge? Listening to truth, not fear.

> *Your affirmation:* I give my emotions the space they need. I take grounded action from a place of discernment and clarity. I am an exceptional listener, and I use this strength to my advantage. I hear what I need to and trust my perception of what's really going on.

If you are a Leo sun sign with Mercury in Cancer, your bold and brave sun sign disposition is accompanied by impeccable sensitivity. You're caring and sensitive with sincere emotional intelligence.

> *Your affirmation:* I leverage my sensitivity and use it to my advantage as I pursue my dreams, goals, and desires. As I nurture myself, I nurture others. My spiritual growth helps me reach my life goals.

Mercury in Leo ♌

If Mercury traveled in the sign of Leo (fixed fire) at the time of your birth, you have a Cancer, Leo, or Virgo sun sign.

Mercury in Leo gives you a propensity toward deep self-expression, leadership, and encouragement of others. You have a commanding voice and mind. And while it's true that you can seem a bit dramatic, in reality you just have incredible passion.

If you are a Cancer sun sign with Mercury in Leo, your sensitive and caring nature takes on a bold and commanding presence.

> *Your affirmation:* I embrace my creative flow by staying aligned with what inspires me. I see my sensitivity as a gift and use it to

unlock my creative magic. I am upbeat, determined, and aware, and I use this on behalf of reaching my goals.

If you are a Leo sun sign with Mercury in Leo, you have to own the right to shine. Your contagious enthusiasm and positive vibes easily uplift others. And you get bonus points for being wicked awesome at manifesting.

Your affirmation: As a leader, I am here to inspire others. I leverage my creativity on behalf of uplifting others. It is safe for me to be seen. I embrace visibility as a part of my path.

If you are a Virgo sun sign with Mercury in Leo, you have an eye for detail but a voice for positivity. With ease and grace you encourage others to do and be their best.

Your affirmation: I inspire and innovate on behalf of being in service to others. When I align with my truth, true inspiration leads me forward. I am here to serve.

Mercury in Virgo ♍

If Mercury traveled in the sign of Virgo (mutable earth) at the time of your birth, you have a Leo, Virgo, or Libra sun sign.

With Mercury, the planet that rules communication, in fastidious, detail-oriented Virgo, you have the upper hand when it comes to precision, technical know-how, and a service-driven heart.

If you are a Leo sun sign with Mercury in Virgo, you have, at your best, a propensity toward what Robert K. Greenleaf coined "servant leadership": leadership that focuses on making sure other people's highest priorities are being served.

Your affirmation: I am service driven and devoted. Self-love strengthens my ability to inspire and uplift others. I focus on progress, not perfection, in order to have optimal impact. I am here to catalyze creativity.

If you are a Virgo sun sign with Mercury in Virgo, you have a deep capacity for precision. Details are your specialty. When it comes to focusing and delivering, you do what you love with razor-blade sharpness.

Your affirmation: I value my attention to detail. I am precise and thorough in my thinking. I stay mindful of my tendency to be critical, of both myself and others. I speak to myself with kindness, and I prioritize compassion when relating to others.

If you are a Libra sun sign with Mercury in Virgo, you have a propensity for balance but an eye for detail. You know how to prioritize the needs of others without abandoning yourself.

Your affirmation: I eloquently ask for what I need. I source my sense of safety and security from within myself. I am adept at meeting my needs with balance and grace.

Mercury in Libra ♎

If Mercury traveled in the sign of Libra (cardinal air) at the time of your birth, you have a Virgo, Libra, or Scorpio sun sign.

With the planet of communication in Venus's domain, loving language comes easy for you. You have a natural propensity toward fairness, but it's important to stay mindful of your people-pleasing tendencies.

If you are a Virgo sun sign with Mercury in Libra, you have an eye for detail, a nose for beauty, and a heart for justice. You know how to bring things back into balance. Yet you can be a bit critical too. While, yes, you want to be "fair," you can also make decisions to please others, which, if left unchecked, can lead to resentment.

Your affirmation: I keep my eyes on the details and my heart on my expansive vision. I allow others to support me. Love inspires and uplifts all that I do and all that I am. I excel at making beauty manifest.

If you are a Libra sun sign with Mercury in Libra, you are fair and balanced in your assessments and have the capacity to speak your mind with brilliance. Learning how to disappoint others gracefully remains your growing edge.

Your affirmation: I live in harmony with the seasonal, hormonal, celestial rhythms that guide my life. I can easily and effortlessly say no, hold my boundaries, and prioritize my deepest needs.

If you are a Scorpio sun sign with Mercury in Libra, you bring beauty and light to darkness. Your justice-driven nature knows how to midwife the truth with sincere grace.

Your affirmation: I am grateful for who I am today, and I love who I am becoming. I live in harmony with my truth. I under-stand what I need, and I know how to ask for it.

Mercury in Scorpio ♏

If Mercury traveled in the sign of Scorpio (fixed water) at the time of your birth, you have a Libra, Scorpio, or Sagittarius sun sign.

With Mercury in "Go deep or go home" Scorpio, introspective, intuitive thinking comes naturally to you. You don't shy away from the truth. Most importantly, you know how to keep a secret. You are trustworthy.

If you are a Libra sun sign with Mercury in Scorpio, your zone of genius lies in relationships. You excel at intimacy. Beyond that, your intuitive capacity is extremely strong. While at times you may feel indecisive, when you trust your gut, you win.

Your affirmation: My intuition guides me expertly, and I listen to it without question. I leverage my emotional intelligence in all aspects of my life, especially my relationships. I know how to be there for others, and for myself too.

If you are a Scorpio sun sign with Mercury in Scorpio, you have a capacity to see, hear, and "know" the truth. You excel when it comes to getting to the bottom of what's actually happening.

Your affirmation: I can trust my intuition and my innate knowing. My determined nature enables me to get what I want. I remain flexible and flow with life.

If you are a Sagittarius sun sign with Mercury in Scorpio, you have an adventurous spirit but a serious mind. Yes, you want freedom, but even more, you want the truth.

Your affirmation: I am not afraid to do the work. My freedom comes through my commitment. I am resilient and strong.

Mercury in Sagittarius ♐

If Mercury traveled in the sign of Sagittarius (mutable fire) at the time of your birth, you have a Scorpio, Sagittarius, or Capricorn sun sign.

With the planet of communication in the bold and blunt sign of Sagittarius, your contagious optimism expresses itself. Yet your untamed honesty, however well intended, can push people harder than they're ready to be pushed.

If you are a Scorpio sun sign with Mercury in Sagittarius, you have an interesting dichotomy. On the one hand, you are introspective and maybe even introverted, but on the other hand, you aren't afraid to speak your truth.

Your affirmation: I am insightful and unafraid to speak my truth, but I do so with patience and tact. I allow my optimism to guide me. I am courageous.

If you are a Sagittarius sun sign with Mercury in Sagittarius, you are bold, blunt, honest, and to the point.

Your affirmation: I embrace my fire, my passion, and my ability to say it like it is. I am courageous and kind. I allow myself to be assertive. I am in touch with how I am feeling, and I can communicate on my behalf without threatening the integrity of others.

If you are a Capricorn sun sign with Mercury in Sagittarius, your hardworking nature benefits from the bon vivant influence that Mercury in Sagittarius brings. The saying "Work hard and play hard" suits your nature.

Your affirmation: I embrace personal mastery on my path of actualizing my highest destiny. I am guided by my vision. I always trust my gut. I am certain of the capacity to succeed.

Mercury in Capricorn ♑

If Mercury traveled in the sign of Capricorn (cardinal earth) at the time of your birth, you have a Sagittarius, Capricorn, or Aquarius sun sign.

With Mercury in Capricorn you favor structure, order, and pragmatism. That doesn't mean you shy away from magic, though; magic just needs to make sense.

If you are a Sagittarius sun sign with Mercury in Capricorn, you are driven by an incredible sense of freedom, but you have a healthy sense of responsibility.

Your affirmation: I am unafraid of hard work, but I understand my self-worth doesn't stem from accomplishment. I take time to pause, reflect, and grow. I source my power from who I am, not what I do.

If you are a Capricorn sun sign with Mercury in Capricorn, you are driven, results oriented, and not afraid of rolling up your sleeves to get work done. Capable and competent, your growing edge remains having a bit of fun.

Your affirmation: Genius is knowing the right use of my work ethic. Just because I can doesn't mean I have to. I exercise discernment and discretion when it comes to saying yes. I have healthy boundaries.

If you are an Aquarius sun sign with Mercury in Capricorn, you have an adventurous spirit but a traditional approach to getting things done. You preserve what's working as you strive to make things better.

Your affirmation: I open my mind to new ideas and possibilities. I love to experiment. I embrace the unknown with confidence.

Mercury in Aquarius ♒

If Mercury traveled in the sign of Aquarius (fixed air) at the time of your birth, you have a Capricorn, Aquarius, or Pisces sun sign.

With Mercury in Aquarius, your quick-witted mind has both intellectual agility and the ability to discern the most efficient path toward your future. You might not always fit in, but then again, you're not supposed to.

If you are a Capricorn sun sign with Mercury in Aquarius, you have a deep respect for tradition, but no time for antiquated practices. Your work ethic serves your progressive ideas. You are here to disrupt the status quo.

Your affirmation: I express my thoughts clearly and coherently. I trust my ideas and my intuition. I am a visionary leader. I am not afraid to speak my mind.

If you are an Aquarius sun sign with Mercury in Aquarius, you have an eye for detail and an eye for design. You embody a balance between forward-thinking ideas and smart, intuitive insight.

Your affirmation: I trust my ideas. I am often ahead of my time, and that's awesome. I grant myself permission to be different.

If you are a Pisces sun sign with Mercury in Aquarius, you embody the perfect blend of emotional intelligence and intuition with original thinking. You have the ideal mix of mental agility and spiritual awareness.

Your affirmation: I can trust my intuition and lean into my empathy as a superpower. I know I am ahead of my time and also a leader.

Mercury in Pisces ♓

If Mercury traveled in the sign of Pisces (mutable water) at the time of your birth, you have an Aquarius, Pisces, or Aries sun sign.

With Mercury in Pisces you have an incredibly intuitive sensibility. You excel at listening and likely even have a poetic way of speaking. You feel before you speak, which means you are intentional with your words.

If you are an Aquarius sun sign with Mercury in Pisces, you have an astute intellect and stealth intuition. Despite being an air sun sign, and at times disconnected from your emotional body, you can express your emotions beautifully by tuning in to how you feel.

Your affirmation: I utilize my gift of perception and my ability to access my emotions to make the changes I most desire and live my best life.

If you are a Pisces sun sign with Mercury in Pisces, you have an incredible capacity to dream, feel, and create. While there's often a desire to escape or check out, by staying disciplined and focused, you can cultivate your dreams. You are a healer.

Your affirmation: I hone my staying power, see my dreams to fruition, and bring healing to the world.

If you are an Aries sun sign with Mercury in Pisces, you have an empathetic heart, but you aren't afraid to ask for what you need. Given your sensitive nature, you can anticipate the needs of others when you communicate. That said, be certain to honor your personal needs too.

Your affirmation: My emotional intelligence guides me as I leverage my capacity to be assertive with my words and ask for what I need. I am comfortable with being both empathetic and assertive. As I ask, so too shall I receive, even if it means being radically uncomfortable and patient in the process.

Mercury in Retrograde (*Rest easy, there's no need to dread!*)

The planet Mercury is linked, mythologically, to the Greek god Hermes, whose story is especially important when discussing Mercury retrograde.

Having won favor with Zeus soon after his birth, Hermes was granted the role of messenger god. Adorned with a winged hat and winged sandals, he also wore a cape to conceal his magic tricks. He was responsible for putting words on the tongues of wily politicians and well-meaning merchants alike. He also ushered the dead into the underworld, and others to Olympus, where the gods lived. Hermes was the only god who could easily traverse the boundaries between Earth, Olympus, and Hades.

We see the clever, yet wily and somewhat tricksterlike nature of Hermes most clearly reflected in the planet Mercury when it's in retrograde. I believe this is something we can, and should, not only enjoy, but also use to our advantage.

Mercury goes retrograde three times a year, for about three weeks each time. Retrograde motion is an optical illusion that happens when a planet appears to go backward. During Mercury retrograde, we can experience feeling like we've been "tricked." However, we can also experience illusions falling away, as we develop a deeper connection to our truth within.

Mercury retrograde is a time to shift speeds and recalibrate. While, yes, snafus may happen, Mercury retrograde invites us to check our hustle at the door, review where we've just been, find the flaw, and rethink our approach. It's when the universe yells, "Plot twist!" and asks us to rethink our perspective, work, and agenda.

While Mercury retrograde often isn't a great time to launch or initiate a big project, it's not a time to halt forward motion either. Instead, we can get ourselves unstuck and make critical shifts to our thinking and our perception. By following our gut instinct and cleaning up issues from the past, we align more with the present—and obtain clear directives on what to execute next.

Ritual: Leverage the Rhythm of the Moon

Ellen Langer, who is a leading pioneer in the mindfulness movement, has researched mindfulness without meditation for well over thirty years. She teaches that we can strengthen our mindfulness, without meditating, by practicing the art of "drawing novel distinctions."[8] By working with moon phases and signs, you can stay super mindful, drawing novel distinctions each day. In doing so, you will also build your own relationship with the rhythm of the moon, learn how to shift a core belief, and fortify your well-being.

Go to JenniferRacioppi.com/resources and download the free *Cosmic Health* ebook. In it you will find a moon journal complete with ritual instructions.

Now that we've taken a deeper look at mindset and Mercury, next we'll explore the role of our passion and values, as well as the planet Venus.

CHAPTER 9

Venus

Beauty, Love, and Body — Harnessing Your Power

Goddess of love, sensuality, fertility, procreation — and special protectress of kings, invoked in war and politics — Inanna, the Sumerian goddess, ruled over all of these aspects of our nature and our world.

As the divine representation of pure, raw feminine power — *not* marriage or motherhood — Inanna used her intelligence, beauty, and wiles to manipulate, endear, and pursue her considerable ambitions. Both ruthless and loving, aggressive and receptive, she was viewed as an equal to men, rather than their subject or victim.

In a human age when women are chastised and ridiculed for claiming the true breadth and depth of our multifaceted nature, we can look to goddesses like Inanna, who embodied the traits of Aphrodite (beauty, receptivity) and Athena (war, power), to create a more comprehensive relationship with the vast power that comes from the creatrix inside us.

In this process of realizing the full range of our potential, astrologically we look to the planet Venus, who, like Inanna, embodies both what she values and the will to fight for it — love as well as war. In claiming these equally essential parts of ourselves, we become the doting lover *and* the unapologetic warrior, the endearing nurturer *and* the almighty protectress, the indulgent hedonist *and* the disciplined go-getter.

In this chapter, we'll look more deeply at the two sides of this primal, empowering energy, which is present in all humans. Then we'll integrate our natal Venus placement to orient ourselves toward this deeper, often only partially developed part of ourselves.

Overwriting Modern-Day Rules

Stay busy. Think positive. Nurture and love, but always for the sake of others. As a rule, keep moving and steer clear of the depths.

We internalize these messages from a young age and grow into productive, ambitious adults who are always busy yet often lack the time and interpersonal connection required to cultivate and pursue our true passions. As women, we are taught to embody love and nurturing, only to be shamed and blamed for claiming its equally empowering counterbalance: the will to fight for what and whom we love.

Disconnected from the true breadth of our nature, we seek fulfillment elsewhere, substituting sugar for sweetness, overwork and overcommitment for a deeper connection to ourselves and others. Detached from our own true value, we engage in tit-for-tat relationships that leave us feeling like we are on the hook for yet another obligation. This all creates so much activity, so much sheer busyness, that we forsake simple pleasures like sitting down at the table long enough to savor a home-cooked meal.

On top of this, we each inhabit a body that, at times, seems precariously vulnerable and out of our control. If that body identifies as female, we feel this vulnerability even more acutely. Any act or expression of pleasure or joy can feel, at best, inconvenient and, at worst, shamefully indulgent, even immoral. Our sexuality is perpetually revered and coveted yet also degraded, even demonized.

Finding our way through this complex, duplicitous culture around what it is to identify as a woman, we further quash our power by saying yes to almost everything—because the minute we say no, we risk being ridiculed or becoming irrelevant. Programmed since a young age to accommodate and acquiesce, we make everyone else feel comfortable. We fit in and avoid making waves. We double down on the emotional labor of raising a family, keeping house, and being the ever-gracious hostess in the office and at home. With so many cultural expectations on our shoulders, we understandably start and end our days feeling more like indentured servants than the representations of the divinity we absolutely are.

To connect with Venus is a deeply empowering yet subversive act. To experience genuine, in-your-bones pleasure is to rewrite the fundamental rules that our society tells us to live by. It's also exactly what we'll accomplish in this chapter.

Reclaiming the Sacred Feminine

The ancients saw the appearance of the morning star as a time to protect and fight for what they loved and desired. The appearance of the evening star, on the other hand, was a time of peace, a chance to nurture, connect, and restore. What they didn't realize was that these two stars were, and remain, one and the same; they are both Venus.

Venus is the cosmic representation of the sacred feminine. As such, we may not be surprised to hear that she represents Aphrodite—a connection to pleasure, embodiment, and collaboration. Yet, as we saw in Inanna, she has a ferocity that is equally important and must also be reclaimed.

While words like "war" imply danger and violence, Venus is not reckless. Instead, she encompasses our visceral power to seek what we most desire, to fight for what and whom we love, and to defend our right to embody the duality of the lover/nurturer and the warrior inside each of us.

Since our male-centric culture could only exist if women occupied a subservient and submissive role, owning the true range of our Venusian nature has been taboo. And so here we are, several millennia later, still attempting to reclaim the full scope of our essence. Yet, in doing so, we ignite the passion, perseverance, and grit to embody our ferocity, enabling us to conjure the life we most desire to live. Cosmic health stems from an unbridled connection to this untamed fervor inside us. Let's begin by looking at both sides of Venus in more depth, beginning with her pleasure-and-beauty-loving side.

Venus: Ruler of Love, Beauty, Pleasure, and Taste

Anja was an Asian corporate executive living in San Francisco whose hugely successful career had failed to overshadow a deep sense of longing, depletion, and despair. Stressed-out, burnt-out, and increasingly cynical about her future, she yearned for the deep connection of an intimate relationship.

With her natal Venus in Gemini, and several important planets in Taurus, which is ruled by Venus, Anja's chart was profoundly influenced by this planet. Since Venus is associated with pleasure and beauty in their many forms, I suggested that she begin with art to start on her healing journey. While this may seem unrelated to her desire for an intimate relationship, Venus's connection to pleasure is a powerful one. When we allow ourselves to experience even some kinds of pleasure that are deeply nourishing to us, we awaken other Venus-related parts of ourselves.

Amazed that I'd "seen" her long-buried love of art, Anja began opting out of after-work drinks, instead pursuing different opportunities to create, and be exposed to, art. From taking classes to attending art gatherings and more, she began to reclaim a feeling of safety around doing something she neglected.

As time went on, she began to get in touch with new parts of herself, including her desire to launch an art-related business. In addition to that, she got certified as a mindfulness instructor, which became her second passion.

Fast-forward a couple of years. Anja is thriving in her corporate career and both of her passion-driven practices. Having reclaimed self-care and pleasure in her life, she's had a total life transformation. In addition to drinking less and eating more healthfully, she's reconnected with the enjoyment of moving her body through exercise.

Now that she's reawakened her Venus-sourced creative energies and power, she feels happier and more confident. She's also in a committed relationship. That's the power of Venus. When we can capitalize on the raw power she bestows upon us, our life mirrors our deepest desires and values.

Undoing the Spell of Pleasure Suppression

In order to inhabit the full scope of our Venus — and the cosmic representation of our multifaceted nature — we need to be able to indulge our inherent need for healthy pleasure and play. While we'll explore the role of both next, first we need to address the cultural spell that's been cast around accommodating our basic need for fun, especially when it's primal in nature.

Women have long been thought of as temptresses who lure men to indulge their carnal desires. While this and many other dances of seduction are natural and healthy, in the role of seductress, women have been portrayed in a negative, even demonic, light. The underlying message has been: to desire is normal and acceptable...as long as you were born male. Even in our "modern" day and age, women who feel, much less express, lust and desire are often cast as whores, harlots, cheaters, and other kinds of "loose" women.

Underlying this double standard is the cultural belief that women who unapologetically pursue and indulge in pleasure are somehow flawed — selfish, immoral, and/or lacking in intelligence, to name just a few of the misperceptions that float around. This idea dates back to many different periods in history, including the time of the Puritans, who rejected our basic human need for pleasure in any form, especially when it was carnal.

Since these beliefs are commonplace among women and all humans, they often affect how willing women are to indulge in pleasure. Lacking in body confidence because we — and nearly every other woman on the planet! — don't live up to impossible standards around the "perfect body," we may inhibit ourselves sexually or engage in unhealthy relationships with other sensual indulgences, like food or alcohol.

In order to correct this balance and put pleasure and play in the more central role they deserve in our lives, we first have to begin detaching from the shame that's been placed on our desire and our need for carnal and sensual pleasure. Instead, we need to give ourselves permission to explore and experience this essential part of ourselves and our power.

Pleasure and Play: Tools of Resilience

Engaging unapologetically in pleasure, play, indulgence — whatever comes to mind when you think of the good life — is also important because it amplifies stress recovery and is therefore central to our health and vitality.

Remember, stress is not inherently bad. The emotions we feel and the body's responses to them serve as data points, signaling intuitive and subconscious understanding that (often) guides us in the right direction. Acute stress that feels depleting — like, say, working so late that we skimp on sleep — shows us what needs to change. When we pay attention and make the necessary adjustments, we become more masterful in our lives and enhance our well-being.

When most of us think of stress, we immediately go negative. However understandable, science confirms that our mindset around stress has a significant impact on how we experience it. Intentionally maintaining a positive mindset around stress does wonders for our health. In fact, finding the opportunity in stress enhances our resilience.[1]

This, however, doesn't mean staying positive at all costs. Or taking on a "good vibes only" mindset, or trying to "love and light" our way through the inevitability of life-defining hardships. Rather, it means facing the conditions that are creating stress with absolute honesty and a resilient mindset.

On top of that, the world overemphasizes productivity, immediacy, and time scarcity. Given that overwhelming reality, it's all too easy to overlook how much stress we're really under. When we don't meet challenges with a resilient mindset and make appropriate behavior change(s), we get trapped in a negative stress spiral. When that happens, the body goes into fight-or-flight mode, releasing norepinephrine and epinephrine to kick us into high gear. This hormonal stress overload can be damaging when it becomes long-lasting, especially if it's not followed by adequate recovery.

While we can't always control how much stress we're under and how we respond to it, we can offset it with pleasure, play, rest, and social connection. When we experience pleasure, helpful secretions—endorphins as well as feel-good hormones like oxytocin—are released in the body, boosting our immune response and ushering in a state of euphoria. On a biological level, we're then better equipped to manage stress, bond with others, trust others, and calm our overtaxed nervous system.

Play has a similar effect on the body and the mind. Dr. Stuart Brown, founder of the National Institute for Play and author of the national bestseller *Play: How It Shapes the Brain, Opens the Imagination, and Invigorates the Soul*, has spent decades studying people's relationships with play. His research has unearthed a strong correlation between play and successful life outcomes. In the context of Venus, play is anything that allows us to engage a healthy sense of mischief. That might mean getting messy in the garden or with an art project, being spontaneous, taking a personal day to play hooky, role-playing in bed, making daring fashion choices—the list goes on. According to Dr. Brown, play puts us in an alternative state that overrides other natural tendencies, including the stress response, and encourages us to explore possibilities and potential. Play also helps us develop empathy and mental flexibility, key skills for navigating a forever-changing, often-stressful world.

Like our emotions, which may get swept aside or wrapped up in an indistinguishable ball of confusion, what we enjoy or truly find fun can also seem hard to figure out. More often than not we've been taught to go along to get along, align with others to feel safe, and resort to codependency. Overworking, too, may leave us disconnected from our joy and uncertain where to find it. Body image issues and addictions also tend to rob us of our vitality; weeks, years, even decades can slip through our hands without us prioritizing our own joy and pleasure.

PLEASURE OR AN ESCAPE?

As with everything, it's important to notice the shadow side of pleasure and play.

One study from the University of Geneva found that stress triggers the body to desire and pursue pleasurable activities that give us a quick and easy boost, like eating sweets. Unfortunately, these activities don't provide enough pleasure to offset stress. Nor do they change our physiology in any positive, enduring ways.[2]

When a pleasurable activity perpetually keeps you from confronting and dealing with challenges and stresses in your life, it's an unhealthy indulgence rather than one that optimizes resilience.

Stay mindful of depriving yourself of the power of facing your stress and pain. You don't need to mask your feelings. You are strong enough to be with them and take the stressors of your life head-on.

Ready to Experiment with Pleasure and Play?

Sometimes the hardest step to take is the first one. Here are some ways to explore bringing more pleasure and play into your life:

- Get wild with music and dancing; go to a concert.
- Be silly and childlike; spend time around kids and/or pets; let your younger self out.

- Embrace gutsiness; find your moxie.
- Get together with your favorite people.
- Engage in a pleasurable, mindful activity, like reading or spending time in nature.

Another pleasurable activity? *Sex.* Sexuality is one path to reacquaint yourself with what feels good, and self-pleasure is a necessary and healthy part of self-care. The health benefits of sex go beyond just feeling good and releasing endorphins. Sexual pleasure boosts the creation of protective antibodies—an immune response that keeps harmful bacteria, viruses, and other germs at bay. Sexual activity has also been shown to lower systolic blood pressure; balance hormone levels; reduce the risk of heart disease, osteoporosis, and prostate cancer; induce relaxation and sleepiness; and enhance memory and analytical thinking.[3]

Venus, Goddess of War, Manipulation, and Conflict

Anja's story shows us how embodying the pleasure-loving side of Venus can help us to thrive throughout our lives. Now we'll examine what happens when we deny Venus's other side—the protector and the warrior.

When I first met Regina, a white woman living in Brooklyn, New York, she felt conflicted, angry, and increasingly hopeless about her career. A married mom with her own business, she had enjoyed some success but still felt profoundly under-realized. For years she'd yearned to launch a side business helping women awaken their creativity. She also had long wanted to complete the novel she'd spent countless hours writing.

While she was passionate about achieving these goals, every time she focused more energy in one of these areas, she'd begin to feel foolish and unworthy. She'd then return her attention to her existing business and resign herself to the belief that she'd never accomplish anything beyond that.

Looking at Regina's chart, I was struck by Venus's pivotal role. Regina had been born on a new moon, and her sun, moon, and Venus were all conjoined in Leo. It's a special position for Venus, and also one that gives Venus a substantial influence over her identity and life.

With so much Leo in her chart, Regina has a deep need to be seen, yet her existing business and work required the opposite — that she *not* be visible. To embody her Leo-infused Venus placement, she also needed to claim the true depth and breadth of her creativity, which was central to her work but also something she hadn't yet allowed herself to unleash fully in her business or her life.

As we began to explore how this tension was playing out in her life, she got quiet. Her hesitation felt heavy and deep-seated. As soon as she spoke, tears began streaming down her face. For decades she'd been avoiding the pain she'd felt growing up, being shamed from a young age for daring to stand out, speak up, and express herself creatively. She was, by nature, a bold, brave soul who'd been taught early that it was shameful to attract attention in overt ways. Afraid of being hurt further, she had learned how to hide in plain sight, tamping down her deep need to express her creativity with the flair and abandon it demanded. This had created a lot of self-doubt, shame, and anger, which sometimes affected her marriage and her parenting in ways that only magnified her shame.

As she began to understand and reconnect with the different manifestations of her Venus placement, Regina realized that she'd been using her Venus warrior spirit to protect and empower others — her clients as well as her son and her husband, both creative souls themselves — but rarely herself. It was time for her to use her inner Venusian warrior in service of her own well-being and happiness. That would mean aggressively pursuing her bigger career dreams, even when they seemed hopeless. On a deeper level, she also needed to address core wounds around reclaiming her creativity and her worth.

It's important to note that women like Regina often experience these kinds of emotional wounds in their body, especially when Venus is involved. Regina was an exception to this rule, partly because of her long-standing healthy habits, which included exercising often and emphasizing whole, nourishing foods. She'd stuck with these habits to feel her best, as she knew she needed them in order to realize her potential.

When I saw Regina a few months later, she looked a little different. Her fingernails were a cool shade of dark green, she'd changed her hair slightly, and she was wearing chunky jewelry with a bold-colored top. She talked about how she'd been allowing herself to have fun with fashion again, which had been a secret passion of hers since childhood (and one that's very much in alignment for anyone with that much Leo in her chart). She was also showing up differently in her friendships with women, as her fun-loving, untamed self, and feeling more connected to herself and them as a result. She'd begun creating an entirely new business too, making sure to infuse her creative flair into the brand's DNA from day one. While these changes were all relatively new, she couldn't say enough about how monumental they were. She was sleeping better, having more fun with her husband and son, and opening up to an entirely new realm of creative self-expression in her life and her work.

Venus and Aligning with Your Values

In reminding us that, beyond engaging in healthy pleasure, we must strive to live in sync with our values, Venus empowers us at the deepest level to let loose our full and multifaceted nature. In this way, Venus guards us against some of the most challenging and debilitating stress we can experience in life—the stress of living out of alignment with our core values. You know what I'm talking about, right? For Regina, it showed up as not honoring her creativity. Most of us experience this imbalance in our lives. Yearning to fit in or achieve or be accepted, we betray ourselves at our core, committing to a life that doesn't represent our truth. That generates chronic stress that's both hard to live with and hard to recover from.

We may also feel out of alignment when we seek compromise in order to reconcile competing values. Many women experience this as the tension between the many roles we play: mom and professional, partner and daughter of aging parents, community leader and spiritual seeker. All of these roles require ongoing commitment and presence; as one example, you can attend your business meeting or your child's school event, but not both at the same time. I experienced a similar but different compromise in the aftermath of my osteoporosis diagnosis. I'd long focused on living a cruelty-free life by not eating animal protein, yet my diagnosis highlighted that I was critically protein deficient.

While competing needs and values can leave us feeling cornered, there's *usually* a workable solution. Emma, whom we met in the previous chapter, is a great example. With a desire to remain true to her gutsy and adventurous self, she unpacked the misbelief that taking care of herself would lead her to become self-centered and superficial, dimming her moxie and joy. She also eliminated the nighttime snacking that had led to her feeling low body confidence and haunted by a habit. Once she tended to the belief that she needed the candy to cope, because she was really afraid to shine, she made the changes necessary to kick the habit that tormented her for almost twenty years. She realized that she could experience pleasure from food *and* feel good in her own skin. At that point, she was free to live in fuller alignment with all of her values.

That's important because in order to experience our most radiant cosmic health, we must connect our values to our goals. When we do this, we're empowered to take inspired action that feeds us on every level. We also have the courage to engage in healthy risk-taking. When we skip over this all-important step and only play it safe, our vitality suffers. Living in mediocrity is a signal to recalibrate with the core values that ignite our most basic desire for well-being. By unleashing and embracing the full range of our Venusian essence, we become fiercely courageous, able to conjure miracles.

Venus in Your Natal Chart: Putting It to Work for You

Venus rules the zodiac signs Taurus and Libra. The position of Venus in your natal chart reveals how you interact with others and what you attract in terms of your personal relationships and material possessions. The sign that Venus occupies indicates the range of how she expresses herself in your chart. The house she shows up in identifies the part of your life that she most strongly influences.

Venus in Aries ♈: Venus in this cardinal fire sign is not afraid to go after what she wants. Think Miranda Priestly, Meryl Streep's character in *The Devil Wears Prada,* or Buffy the Vampire Slayer. Knowing what you most want, defining what you love and why you love it, is all you need to conquer and manifest your desires.

Venus in Taurus ♉: This is one of Venus's most beloved positions. Since Venus rules Taurus (fixed earth), you have an innate knack for pleasure. Nourishment and sensuality connect you to your divinity. Think delicious sensual food, a hot bath, a beautiful walk in nature. To unlock Venus's powers, you need to take it slow and enjoy the little things.

Venus in Gemini ♊: Travel, networking, stimulating adventures—Venus in this mutable air sign seeks to make the most of Gemini's fast-moving energy by being light, breezy, and easy, not heavy or deep. Your social charms are among your greatest powers, and you are adept at sharing information. It's important for you to write, even if just in a journal.

Venus in Cancer ♋: Venus in this cardinal water sign shines in making others feel welcome and nurtured. Cancer is a food-oriented sign, so hosting dinner parties might just be your sweet spot. You bond with people deeply and delight in caring for them. You have incredible emotional grace. Capitalize on this, and use it to your advantage by nurturing your emotional intelligence.

Venus in Leo ♌: Venus in this fixed fire sign of expression underscores the importance of giving voice to your instinct for pleasure and play, which are nonnegotiable for you. Entertaining and enjoying social activities serves you well, as does creative expression in its many forms. Be bold and brave. Be you.

Venus in Virgo ♍: With Venus in the mutable earth sign of the maiden, you have the capacity to love with the purest of devotion. For you, pleasure may come in the form of health routines or a disciplined practice. Play frees you to enjoy what naturally nourishes you. You embody the priestess archetype.

Venus in Libra ♎: Venus in the cardinal air sign of the scales lends itself to balance, harmony, and justice. Your sense of style, both in fashion and home décor, is off the charts. Partnership is important to you, but don't sell yourself short. Make sure it's true love — the right person — rather than infatuation or your deep yearning to have "the one."

Venus in Scorpio ♏: With Venus in this fixed water sign, you navigate taboo topics like none other. With an inclination toward mystery, your natural investigative qualities demand emotional depth and intimacy. You embody intensity and a need for sensuality, yet you also tend toward possessiveness.

Venus in Sagittarius ♐: With Venus in the mutable fire sign of the archer, you aim at what you love. Always dreaming of the next open road, you crave adventure and fun. You're naturally outgoing and social, and don't like relationships that limit or challenge your freedom. For those reasons, you may choose to remain single or partner up later in life, but when you love, you love big.

Venus in Capricorn ♑: With Venus in the cardinal earth sign of the sea goat, you're innately drawn to structure, a dedicated work ethic, and purposeful devotion. You have great taste, and you're fiercely loyal to those you love and respect. You stoically show up on behalf of your values.

Venus in Aquarius ♒: With Venus in the fixed air sign of the water bearer, you're naturally innovative. You love your freedom and are not always inclined toward traditional relationships. More open than most to the unconventional, you seek to explore your many interests. As a mover and shaker, your visionary nature puts you in a position of leadership.

Venus in Pisces ♓: When the goddess of pleasure finds her way into the mutable water sign of the fish, she embodies sensitivity and romance. Drawn toward communion with source and spirituality, you are well served by embracing the arts. Music, theater, photography, and dance all unleash a sense of sensuality and pleasure in your life. Just beware of your inclination toward escapism.

Venus in Retrograde

From our perspective on Earth, Venus can move from sign to sign in three to four weeks or spend as long as four months in a single sign due to her retrograde motion. Venus goes retrograde every eighteen months, for approximately forty days.

We've already looked at how Venus represents the two sides of the sacred feminine. When she's positioned as the evening star, she's known as Venus Hesperus, the embodiment of passion and allure in their most benevolent forms. When Venus rises in the east with the sun, she is at her brightest, a warrior known as Venus Lucifer, bearer of light. She switches between her two sides every nine months. During her retrograde, she moves from her evening star into her morning star position.

In retrograde, Venus is energetically called back to her internal wildness to reclaim her worth and what has been lost within. After retreating to the underworld to reexamine who she is, who she loves, and what she values, she's reignited. And she's ready to kick some ass.

During her retrograde period, Venus asks you to enter into your own underworld and face the sides of yourself that you might not regularly identify with: your rage, anger, and jealousy. Here your shadow begs for attention and healing. This retrograde transit may highlight how you relate to your values, relationships, body, money, friendships, sexuality, fertility, and sensuality—all of which fall under Venus's domain. How a given retrograde affects you personally depends on the sign the retrograde happens in and your personal chart.

In retrograde, Venus can help you excavate an area where you have given away your power or betrayed a core value. While this asks you to go deep into areas you may prefer to avoid, it can also create an opportunity to reclaim tremendous strength, personal agency, and healing momentum.

Venus retrograde is a time to recommit to your true essence and values.

Venus Ritual: Owning the Warrior and the Lover

This is a ritual to help you conjure and experience the force of love in your life. The most auspicious times for this ritual are when there's a new or full moon in Libra or Taurus (Venus rules them both). Or when she transitions the time of day she rises, which happens every nine months. In this ritual, we embrace the two sides of Venus: her morning star position, where Venus heralds the journey of going after her desires, and her evening star position, where she basks in pleasure and embodies the richness of earthly delights.

Before beginning this ritual, you may want to repeat the cosmic bath in the Full Moon Ritual (see chapter 5). That will help to cleanse and purify your energy, but it's not a required step; this ritual is powerful regardless.

To begin this ritual, you need some simple items:

- Three candles: one that symbolizes your warrior spirit, another that symbolizes your goddess spirit, and a third that represents the union of the two. The colors, shapes, and sizes of the candles are up to you.

- One small bowl of water
- A pinch of salt
- Music — just one song — that elevates you

When you're ready, sit at your altar or on a meditation cushion. Mix the salt and water together. As you do this, you're creating a powerful blend of the elements of earth and water that, when combined, promote the healing properties of both these elements.

Sprinkle this salt water on your altar or simply dip your fingers into the bowl and then put a dab of salt water at the point between your brows, also known as your third eye.

Now take a seated position. Gently lower your eyelids and connect with your inner cosmos, the universe within. Once you feel that connection, begin to feel your power expand. Take a moment to imagine Venus in her morning star position. There she is, fiery, motivated, and capable of defending what and whom she loves. Light the candle that connects to Venus in this warrior position.

When you are ready, connect with Venus in her evening star position as she emerges from within you. Here you can bask in the delights of life: pleasure, luxury, joy, receptivity. Light the candle that represents Venus in this position. With both candles burning, feel the totality of Venus's range. She defends *and* she delights.

Then connect with your own range. Your ferocity and your receptivity, your anger and your compassion, your fierce love and your nurturing love. Think of as many opposites as you can to define yourself, then imagine all of these polarities unified by one common value: love. Then light the third candle representing this union.

Think about people, places, moments, and experiences that bring you into the essence of love.

When you are ready, play one song that elevates you even further into the vibration of love. If you feel called to dance, please do.

When you feel complete, come back to your altar and thank Venus. Then extinguish the candles.

CHAPTER 10

Mars

Planet of Action and Motivation

How do we harness the energy and drive to take bold action in our lives? How do we muster the courage to go after our hopes and dreams when it doesn't feel natural or easy?

Many of us have been taught that success and achievement—whether it's with our health, work/career, relationships, or something else—comes from setting goals and relying on discipline, routine, and determination to take the necessary action. While realizing any big goal does often require commitment and consistency, is that really *all* it takes?

Honestly?

To take bold action toward our goals repeatedly, we have to look deeper—at how we gather the will to create movement in our bodies and our lives. Without that essential raw energy and drive to move forward, we stall and get stuck, cycling in and out of positive habits, ultimately falling short of accomplishing our goals.

To experience cosmic health and make the utmost of our healing powers, we need to harness our vigor and our tenacity. We need to conjure and cultivate our passion and fuel our resilience. Doing so aids our ability to create through intention and will, in communion with forces inside and outside ourselves.

Cosmically, Mars drives our propensity toward action and relates to our body's physical energy.

Next we'll look at what prevents us from taking bold action and how we can mobilize our courage and energy. Then we'll use our natal Mars placement to move definitively toward our desires.

Sourcing the Will to Act from Within

What if we could source our most powerful, enduring will to take action toward manifesting our desires not through discipline or determination but through invigoration and purposeful use of power? What if the activation of love and grit is what we need, not dogged discipline alone?

What if realizing our most abundant and fulfilling cosmic health — including making the changes we need to make — is almost like a chain reaction that we can activate by doing something we were literally born to do?

In 2003, John J. Ratey, associate professor of clinical psychiatry at Harvard Medical School, traveled to Naperville, Illinois, to witness how that process was unfolding in the district's grade schools. At a time when most school districts in the US were ranked in tenth to fifteenth place worldwide in math and science, the students in Naperville had scored number one in science and number six in math worldwide.

Interestingly, the students' success was partly the result of the town's K–12 physical education (PE) program. Every day all of the K–12 students were required to attend a forty-five-minute PE class, which focused on increasing students' fitness rather than on developing specific sports skills. As a result, the students' academic performance had skyrocketed.

Dr. Ratey was captivated, well aware that the students' improved academic performance had a lot to do with their required daily physical activity. As he explains in his book *Spark: The Revolutionary New Science of Exercise and the Brain*, rigorous physical exercise does more than burn energy. It turns on the brain, activating the prefrontal cortex (the brain's "CEO," which controls executive functions and impulses), creating neurotransmitters (which affect our mood and emotions), and causing the release of brain-derived neurotrophic factor (BDNF), or as Dr. Ratey calls it, "Miracle-Gro for the brain," a protein that keeps the brain young and staves off age-related cognitive decline.[1]

Excited about the changes that had occurred in the students in Naperville, Dr. Ratey and his team took those findings to schools with students who weren't thriving in an academic setting. One high school in southern Ontario, Canada, began a fitness-based program for a group of students who frequently exhibited disruptive behavior. These were kids with unstable home lives who often got suspended for violating school rules. Within months, their suspensions dropped from ninety-five days down to five days. Those same kids' school attendance also increased. Another school in Charleston, South Carolina, instituted a fitness-based physical education program and saw an 83 percent decrease in discipline problems in the first four months.[2]

If moving our bodies can elevate our cognitive performance, increase our ability to focus, and level out our emotions, what can it do for our cosmic health—and, in turn, our lives?

Exercise Your Body, Power Your Brain (and Soul)

Every morning, my phone would ring. Frank, my personal trainer, would be calling to wake me up. It was usually still dark out, and minutes later I would drag myself to the beach to begin a grueling workout. The overall experience was awesome, brutal, and invigorating all at once; what it did was spark my miracle-making proclivities, ultimately setting my life ablaze on an up-leveled trajectory.

I was at a transitional stage in my life, struggling with depression while also yearning to find my career, work through my emotional baggage, travel around the world, and generally expand and make miracles happen. I'd hired a life coach to kick-start that process, and doing so had led me to reprioritize exercise. Enter Frank and his early morning phone calls to wake me up and get me to meet him for my workout.

We're taught to view exercise as something we do for the body. However, as I experienced, and as Dr. Ratey has spent much of his career teaching, moving the body is at least as beneficial for the brain. In addition to improving cognition, it's one of the most powerful and reliable treatments for depression.

At Duke University, researchers conducted a controlled four-month study of the effects of exercise on older patients suffering from major depression. During the experiment, 156 patients were divided into three groups: one group was given an antidepressant drug; the second group exercised regularly; the third group took the antidepressant and exercised. At the end of four months, the exercise-only group experienced improvements comparable to both other groups. Six months after the study, 8 percent of those who continued to exercise relapsed into depression, whereas 38 percent of the antidepressant-only group and 31 percent of the exercise-and-antidepressant group relapsed into depression.[3]

While there's no denying the important role medication can play in treating depression, I experienced the very real catalytic powers that exercise provides during those months when I worked out with Frank. Weeks into our boot-camp-style sweat sessions, I started feeling a confidence that wasn't just more deeply rooted; it was bolder and braver. I began laying down boundaries with toxic people and influences in my life and prioritizing my dreams, in ways and to an extent that I never had before. I also had more energy, clarity, and focus. I seemed to have more moxie.

While I'd been an athlete throughout high school, my cancer-ridden college years had robbed me of my vitality, my trust in my body, and my ability to exercise. Thanks to Frank and his grueling workouts, I reconnected with this part of myself. After a few weeks of our daily workouts, I felt renewed, like a deeply nourishing fire had been lit inside me, keeping me safe, energized, and empowered.

I loved how strong and integrated my body felt, sure, but what kept me getting up each morning wasn't the physical changes in my body; it was how I felt — emotionally, mentally, and spiritually — as a result of my daily workouts with Frank. Finally, it was clear: my body wasn't irreversibly broken. I could still source my energy and power through action, and I could kick-start that entire process by activating my body. It was like a chain reaction, a spark that was first lit on the physical plane and then spread quickly to my emotions, filling me with a deep faith in my body, myself, and my life. Exercise helped me tap into the passion and intensity of desire I needed to set my miracle-making mojo ablaze.

Feeling more whole than I had in years, I experienced a huge boost in my self-esteem, knowing that moving my body gave me this deep sense of mastery and connectedness with my emotions and my capacities. I could feel better every day, I could use my excitement and creativity to manifest my desires—and it all began with exercise.

Exercising for Mental Health

Walking is the best medicine.
—HIPPOCRATES

Since Hippocrates's time, exercise has somehow become a way to achieve a so-called bikini body when, in fact, as he stated repeatedly throughout his life, it's our most reliable gateway to physical, mental, and emotional well-being. As my teacher Dr. Tal Ben-Shahar often said in his positive psychology lectures, "Not exercising is like taking a depressant."

Kim, a white woman and a professional musician living in New York City, had struggled with anxiety and depression for years when she got pregnant. Concerned how pregnancy would affect her creative process, she began attending daily fitness classes. Very quickly that became a nonnegotiable source of hope and healing in her life. At nine months pregnant, she felt stronger than she ever had. As gratifying as that was, for Kim the emotional recalibration that exercise enabled in her was what kept her going back day after day.

This emotional modulation happens because moving your body triggers a positive neurochemical reaction that allows you to feel more in control, happier, and physically and mentally stronger. Encouraging the release of endorphins, exercise inhibits anxiety reactions and promotes a sense of calm, even euphoria. These naturally occurring chemicals also contribute to sharper cognitive function and memory, warding off age-related mental decline.

Ongoing research also informs us that exercise increases synaptic transmission of monoamines (like epinephrine and serotonin) that can help to counter depression. Separate studies find that consistent exercise protects against the development and relapse of depression; a 2019 Harvard study found that running for fifteen minutes a day or walking for an hour reduces the risk of depression by 26 percent.

MIND-BODY HEALING IN ACTION

Exercise is one of the quickest ways to fuel your body and mind with powerfully positive mojo. Here's additional research linking physical activity to emotional well-being and resilience:

- In a 2014 study on regular exercise and resilience, regular exercisers showed a lesser decline in positive mood after exposure to stress compared to non-exercising participants.[4]
- A study of more than three hundred teachers—a profession known for its high levels of psychological pressure, adversity, and burnout—found that those who engaged more in physical exercise displayed greater levels of psychological resilience. This included recovering from stress, overcoming disappointment, and adapting to new circumstances.[5]
- Researchers Jasper Smits, PhD, and Michael Otto, PhD, found that regular exercise acts as a type of exposure therapy, particularly for those prone to anxiety and heightened stress responses. Because exercise creates physical reactions similar to what we experience during fight-or-flight circumstances (like perspiration and increased heart rate), regular exercise helped participants associate these physiological responses with safety rather than danger.[6]

Beyond its physiological effects, exercise can act as a positive distraction and provide a healthy break from prolonged exposure to stressful circumstances and negative thoughts. It also helps us feel a sense of accomplishment.

If this tribute to exercise doesn't convince you, I will leave you with one last tidbit: physical activity is a natural way to attune yourself to the hustle and flow of life. Exercise both increases your energy level over time and helps you get more restorative sleep at night. From this perspective, movement is less an expenditure of energy and more of an upgrade in your overall ability to perform, thrive, and be well.

ON LOVE, JOY, AND MOVEMENT

What if moving your body does more than improve your mental and physical health? In her inspiring and well-researched book *The Joy of Movement: How Exercise Helps Us Find Happiness, Hope, Connection, and Courage,* Kelly McGonigal, PhD, takes us on a global tour of different cultures and how they use and benefit from movement. Here are a few of my favorite takeaways from her work:

- **The exerciser's "high" makes us more loving.** People who regularly engage in movement long enough to experience the bewitching hormonal cocktail known as the runner's/exerciser's "high" often describe it as a feeling of intense, overwhelming love—for their loved ones, themselves, and the world. That's some beautiful magic!

- **Synchronized group movement fosters collective joy.** Whether it's a rowing club in Canada, group dancing in South America, or exercise classes in California, when we exercise together, we experience communal joy.

> • **Making movement a regular part of your life builds resilience, confidence, and grit.** Those who prioritize movement on a regular basis benefit from more than stronger muscles. Showing up for workouts week after week is linked to an increased ability to bounce back from disappointment and setbacks and to experience greater self-esteem.

Commit to Feeling Amazing

Remember Heather, the business owner who used routine and structure to keep herself energized? Her daily schedule demands a consistently high level of excellence and focus. To stay sharp and feel her best, she goes to the gym every day at 5:30 a.m. Like clockwork, she works out with a trainer two days a week, and on the remaining three weekdays, she reads while on the elliptical. She looks forward to exercising *every day*; it's her time for herself. It also happens to be great for her productivity because it fires up her brain first thing each morning. Starting her day with movement also boosts her energy and leaves her feeling ready to manage the considerable stress and pressure she constantly navigates.

As a Gemini, I tend to need more variability in my schedule, but I too share Heather's, as well as Kim's, commitment to movement. While I often exercise in the morning, sometimes it doesn't fit into my schedule until later in the day. Regardless, I prioritize exercise. It's a crucial part of how I treat osteoporosis. I've made that commitment because when I feel good in my body, I'm physically and mentally stronger. I consistently experience more ease and flow throughout my life, perform better in my work, and feel happier and more confident. I also sleep a lot better. I feel so strongly about the importance of exercise that one of my clients once told me that I should write a blog entitled *You Want to Make More Money? Exercise!* (And she's right!)

While I practice strength training, I often like to run, not because of how fast or far I run—I'm not exceptional in either of those ways—but because of how it makes me feel. A lot of people dislike running, and the good news is there are many different ways to get your heart rate up and your blood pumping. Whichever activities you choose, here are three things to look for in a good workout:

1. **Do you feel your brain breathing?** There's something magical that happens when I'm running and in a good cycle of breath — I can feel the air going through my nasal passages and into the front of my skull. It's as if I can feel my brain breathing, and with that space in my brain, my thoughts naturally soften.

2. **Is your face relaxed?** When I'm in my sweet spot, I begin to feel the skin around my temples and jawline loosen. From there, I pay attention to how free my face feels as I continue to push forward. Is it moving with the pace of my step? If so, that's good. What I look for is deep relaxation of the muscles in my face, particularly around the jawline, where we often hold tension.

3. **How's the quality of your sweat?** There's nothing more gratifying than well-earned sweat! I love feeling it come through my pores and cleanse my skin. When that happens, I know I'm in a good place.

To be clear, exercise is *not* about body size, appearance, or weight loss. It's about making a commitment to feeling amazing every single day.

MEETING YOUR BODY WHERE IT'S AT

Some of us, including myself since my osteoporosis diagnosis, have to moderate exercise for medical reasons. Others can't exercise at all.

While physical therapy, chair yoga, using a resistance band, and/or light weight lifting while seated provide low-impact options for mobility challenges, meeting your body where it's at is the most important step you can take. And sometimes this means staying in bed! Please do not shame yourself for this. Instead, focus on what you can do, and trust that your healing magic is coming exactly as it should even if you can't exercise.

Mars, Planet of Action and War

When we talk about taking action, exercising, and creating movement of any kind in our lives, cosmically we're referring to Mars, the planet of war and action, named after the Roman god of war.

Mars is about dynamic action;[7] it fuels us with the impulse to create momentum and change, and, when necessary, to get angry. While the energy of Mars, if unbridled, can become overly warrior-like — too prone toward action, anger, and aggression — Mars itself plays a crucial role in our ability to generate outcomes and realize goals, including achieving and maintaining cosmic health.

Mars enables us to take action, to forge a new path in spite of the many obstacles we inevitably face. Without Mars, our desires (Venus) and mindset shifts (Mercury) would prove fruitless. However, with Mars, almighty planet of action and war, at our side, we rise, brave and bold, to face adversity with valor and steadfast determination.

In Roman mythology Mars was the second most powerful god, superseded only by Jupiter. As the celebrated protector of Rome,[8] Mars was adorned in shining armor, with power that was known to be formidable, invincible, and magnificent. Calling only the most blessed and able warriors to his "field of renown," Mars deems that to die as his warrior on the battlefield is among the highest of honors.[9]

With Venus, we began to harness the power of our lover/warrior energy. With Mars we take that further, activating our energy and drive through exercise and action, and also by accessing one of our most powerful, yet forbidden, emotions: anger.

How Anger Can Ignite Your Healing Process

On a deeper emotional level, anger is connected to our ability to take action, which is critical to accessing our healing magic, as well as the power of the planet Mars. Especially for women, anger is a taboo emotion, one we're taught not to express, or even feel.

Yet anger's role in our ability to take bold action, heal, and realize our full potential must not be overlooked. Anger, even rage, is intimately connected to our survival instinct. Like love and desire, anger is a primal and necessary emotion. When we're in danger, anger is our signal to fight or flee, and without it, we're unable to defend ourselves. Our anger helps us understand where our boundaries have been violated.

For her 2016 album *Lemonade*, Beyoncé recorded a music video in which she becomes the scorned lover, smashing in car windows with a baseball bat just before cracking the top off a fire hydrant. The album quickly became controversial, partly because it took us through the arc of feminine resurrection, and her anger was a part of that. What if, instead of viewing it as shameful or reprehensible, we could view healthy anger expression as what it is: a catalyst for courage and boldness?

While we're taught to associate anger with causing harm to others, appropriately expressing all of our emotions is essential to our health and well-being. Anger expression is, in fact, a form of catharsis that's critical to our mental and physical well-being. Catharsis allows us to release and purify, which is what Beyoncé does in her music video. She does this *without* hurting anyone, although with some property damage for dramatic, Hollywood-style effect.

One of the reasons we're taught to fear and suppress anger is that it's such a big, overpowering emotion. However, the sheer power of anger is also why it's so important for us to find healthy ways to express it. When we fail to express anger, that tornado of suppressed emotion stays inside us, overpowering our thoughts and other emotions, even hijacking our innate ability to heal. This stifles us.

Expressing anger lightens our cognitive load and gives us a powerful gateway to clarity and a better grasp on grief. Here is just some of the research about the healing power we can access by expressing and releasing anger:

- In a study of more than seven hundred college students, those who reported expressing anger through discussion also reported greater levels of optimism and self-efficacy, compared to those who reported suppressing anger or expressing anger in a blaming way.[10]

- Acknowledging and reflecting on anger can lead to greater self-insight and change. In a study of Russian and American populations, one-third of participants reported that expressing anger helped them better understand their own faults.[11]
- A study conducted by the University of Tennessee found that people who suppressed their anger were more likely to develop cancer, and that continued suppression may contribute to the cancer's progression.[12] Further studies identify suppressed anger as a risk factor for heart disease, colds, flu, skin disease flare-ups, and more.[13]

While anger can be a destructive force, when it's channeled productively, it can motivate us to take greater risks and achieve an important goal. In this way, experiencing our anger can propel us to take action that transforms us, our health, and our lives in the best possible ways.

For all of these reasons, it's incredibly important to pay attention to your anger and to take the time you need to express it in healthy ways. This can look like channeling it creatively by journaling, dancing, or making art. But it can also look like getting political, protesting, screaming behind closed doors, and pounding pillows. Maybe it means talking it out with a friend, or letting someone who hurt you know that they did harm. Or perhaps process it with the support of a licensed therapist. Whatever you choose, know this: by reclaiming your anger, you are taking a meaningful step forward.

Mars in Your Natal Chart: Putting It to Work for You

Mars is the ruler of Aries as well as the co-ruler of Scorpio. In addition to being the start of the zodiacal year, Aries season begins in March, which is named after the planet Mars.

Where Mars is placed in your natal chart reveals how you can assert yourself in a way that feels most natural to you. Your Mars placement also illuminates how you may channel your passions and activism.

Mars in Aries ♈: Mars rules Aries (cardinal fire), so with this placement, you have a natural sense of ambition, drive, and determination. At times this intensity can fuel anger, so finding ways to express and release your emotions remains paramount. Incorporating movement that both challenges and rewards you helps you process emotion. When it comes to working out, prioritize activities that maximize your effort; kickboxing is great for emotional catharsis, but so is dance, cycling, rowing, or jogging. Regardless of what you choose for movement, let it be fun and uplifting.

Mars in Taurus ♉: Mars in Taurus (fixed earth) may mean that you are the type of person who can't be rushed. You take your time and pounce only if or when you are ready, because once you're in, there's no going back. You're incredibly loyal. Consider committing to an exercise routine that helps you feel more embodied, like walking, dance, hiking, or trail running. You do well when you exercise outdoors, so optimize that when weather allows. At times you can resist movement, so please watch out for that. Call yourself out, get an accountability buddy, and by all means, make sure you are exercising regularly, even if that means putting on tunes and dancing in front of the mirror.

Mars in Gemini ♊: With Mars in Gemini (mutable air), you are flexible and curious. You need a wide array of stimulation to keep your mojo rising. To that point, make sure you're exercising your mind as much as your body. Read, network, socialize. With regards to movement, it's oh so important for you to do activities that stimulate your breath and ground you. While you may desire an active nightlife—and yes, going dancing counts as movement—it's also important for you to develop the discipline and rigor of just straight-up exercise. Because Gemini can be a bit here, there, and everywhere, you want to consciously corral your life-force energy and keep your Mars accountable. For you, discipline is everything.

Mars in Cancer ♋: With Mars in Cancer (cardinal water), you have a fierce need to protect what matters. Your emotional depth and breadth are almost unmatched, yet that can also create challenges around setting healthy boundaries. You're innately driven to care for others; it's important to remember to care for yourself. Your job is also to manage moodiness, which may get the best of you at times. When this happens, remember the emotional and medicinal benefits of movement. A morning movement routine will help you enormously. Varying your workouts and working with the phases of the moon will help you to process your emotions in healthy ways.

Mars in Leo ♌: Mars in Leo (fixed fire) infuses you with passion and a powerful and inspiring playfulness. You uplift others in ways that attract attention and elevate your own visibility. Action-oriented by nature, you are the eternal optimist, motivated to have fun and bring more joy to the world. Make sure to focus on movement that you genuinely enjoy, and maybe also something you can wear a fun outfit for. Self-expression is catalytic for you. Think hip-hop dance, high-intensity interval training, or anything action oriented that mobilizes you. On an emotional level, Mars in this sign can be a wee bit dramatic, so beware of getting carried away.

Mars in Virgo ♍: With Mars in Virgo (mutable earth), you are the hardworking hero of any cause you deeply believe in. With your sharp eye for precision and your inclination toward consistency, your innate work ethic guides you. You thrive when dealing with details, but you also may tend toward perfectionism. Instead of going down rabbit holes and splitting hairs about aspects that may not ultimately matter, step back and consider the big picture. For movement, consider Pilates or other precision-oriented practices that combine movement, breath, and alignment. Spending time in nature heals and motivates you. Get outdoors whenever possible.

Mars in Libra ♎: With Mars in Libra (cardinal air), the sign of balance and fairness, your passion for justice inspires you to fight for what you know is right. Your finely attuned aesthetic sensibilities are a gift, enabling you to create unparalleled beauty. Your deep desire for partnership is important but can also leave you vulnerable to getting enmeshed with others. In all of your relationships, make sure to ask for what you need, even when that means rocking the proverbial boat. Learning to say no supports your emotional equilibrium. For you, consider any kind of movement that's accompanied by music, or partnered sports, to bring you back into harmony. If you lose your center, your breath balances you.

Mars in Scorpio ♏: With the planet of action, Mars, in Scorpio (fixed water), a sign he co-rules, your passion is at full throttle. This isn't a mild placement for Mars but rather a call to full-force effort and commitment to depth, intimacy, and sensuality. Follow what naturally turns you on. You're attracted to mystery and the bare, naked truth, but your intensity can overwhelm people. Your aptitude for the noir can lead you too close to the edge at times. When it comes to movement, all of the normal contenders apply, with one qualifier—do *not* override your instincts. Focus on a movement practice that ignites your sacred sexuality to get the most out of your effort. Try classes in hip-hop or even pole dancing.

Mars in Sagittarius ♐: With Mars in Sagittarius (mutable fire), your passionate devotion to freedom, truth, and self-expression is undeniable. A mover and shaker by nature, you are energized by travel. When managing and expressing your emotions, notice your bold and blunt approach. Not everyone is ready for your brand of truth. Aerobic activity is crucial to your well-being; choose a practice that brings a sense of spaciousness to your body and mind, ideally one that resonates philosophically. Whenever possible, emphasize outdoor activities, like hiking, biking, trail running, and winter mountain sports. Vigorous indoor activities like cycling, swimming, and strength training are also favorable.

Mars in Capricorn ♑: Mars does exceptionally well in Capricorn (cardinal earth), blessing you with stamina, determination, and drive. Your grit and deep sense of responsibility fuel your potential to rise to the top. However, you may make things harder than they need to be. Your genius lies in knowing the best use of the inexhaustible work ethic this placement can bring. Spin classes, rowing, weight training, or anything that lets you measure your progress and push your limits keeps you motivated. Restorative activities, like yin yoga, are also an important counterbalance. When managing challenging emotions, you have the courage to face the truth and make it better. Rock on.

Mars in Aquarius ♒: With Mars in Aquarius (fixed air), you are innately mission oriented, fueled by a deep desire to work for the good of the collective. You are adept at digesting the big picture and taking action to realize any vision that aligns with your ideals. For you, mindset is crucial, since your intrinsic motivation demands that your actions reflect your values. Regular, consistent movement of any kind connects you with your higher mind. When dealing with anger or other difficult emotions, understand that it can be hard for you to locate your true emotions, especially anger. Check in with yourself regularly to connect with how you're really feeling.

Mars in Pisces ♓: With Mars in Pisces (mutable water), the sign of dreams, your proverbial get-up-and-go can feel more like get-up-and-go *to bed and dream*. Own the power of your sometimes dreamlike inner world; it's at the core of your deeply spiritual nature. Your capacity for empathy is unmatched. More than most, you bring and create peace where others cannot. On an emotional level, learning how to name your emotions helps you to process them. To inspire yourself to move, keep in mind that music is gold; whenever you can incorporate it into your movement practice, do it. Movement that involves a meditative focus supports you immensely.

Mars in Retrograde

Mars relates to yang energy, which is associated with structure, logic, control, power, assertiveness, and the act of creation. This can show up as your vitality, your will to live, your sex drive, your capacity to weather storms in relationships, and your commitment to career and your life purpose. As you can imagine, when Mars is in a retrograde cycle, which happens roughly once every twenty-six months, lasting from sixty to eighty days, you may enter a time of profound reevaluation.

Mars rules passion and action, so a retrograde cycle dims his energy and power. During Mars retrograde, your gusto may feel out of reach. On a deeper level, Mars retrograde asks you to reassess your mission and goals. Even if it feels tedious, go back over your work and commitments to be sure they accurately reflect you and your desires.

Mars's retrograde may also lower your drive to get a sweat on. If you don't feel like going the extra mile, it's okay, but don't abandon your movement practice.

Mars Ritual: Reclaim the Disavowed

This is a ritual to help you reclaim the healing power of anger as a way to connect to your life vision and goals. You can do this ritual at any time. It's particularly helpful when you feel stifled or upset.

To begin this ritual, you need some simple items:

- One candle that symbolizes your warrior spirit (this can be the same candle you used for your Venus ritual)
- Music — just one song — that connects you to your rage

When you're ready, sit at your altar, gently lower your eyelids, and connect with your inner cosmos, the universe within. Once you feel that connection, begin to feel your power expand. Take a moment and connect to your inner Mars. There he is: intense, demanding, and fierce. Conjuring this side of you, light the candle connecting you to your inner warrior.

Then connect with your own rage. Think about people, places, moments, and experiences that catalyze your anger. What upsets you, ignites you, lights up your ferocity, your anger, *and* your compassion, your fierce love, your passion and intensity? Take a moment to feel these often under-recognized emotions and triggers. Allow yourself to feel!

When you are ready, play one song that allows you to feel angry— like punk rock, heavy metal, or brooding classical music. Whatever it is, just make sure it's dark and stormy. Then get up and dance. As you do, stomp, growl, scream, or whatever else helps you to express your emotions. Fully feel whatever is coming up for you.

When the song is over, come back to your altar and tune in to your body. How does it feel? What sensations are present? Get curious.

Now ask yourself this: *What's something positive I can do with these feelings? How can I channel them toward my creativity? What action do they inspire me to take?* Think about it.

Open your journal and freewrite about how you can channel your emotions toward your own creativity. Don't edit; just let your consciousness stream onto the page.

Once you feel complete with your answer, read it back to yourself out loud. How do you feel? What's coming up for you? Check in with yourself.

Now journal in the same way on this question: *Who do I need to be to make this vision a reality?*

Once you feel complete with your answer, read it back to yourself out loud. How do you feel? What's coming up for you? Check in with yourself.

Finally, ask yourself this: *What's one action I can commit to taking that will bring me closer to my goal?*

In your journal, write out your answer.

Once you are clear, commit to taking this action. Say it out loud. Write it on a piece of paper. Then leave it on your altar.

Extinguish the candle.

CHAPTER 11

Jupiter

Harbinger of Joy and Abundance

What is luck and how can we get more of it? It's a question most of us have asked ourselves at various times in our lives. If we don't see ourselves as one of the "lucky ones," are we eternally doomed, whether in health, love, money, or other life categories?

Now that we've shifted our mindset (Mercury), grounded ourselves in our desires and values (Venus), and sprung into action (Mars), next we'll look at another element of cosmic health: our ability to support and receive grace—also known as luck or blessings—in our lives. In addition to viewing this from a positive psychology standpoint, we'll of course consider it from a cosmic one, via the planet Jupiter.

Aus·pi·cate

My friend Wendy Yalom introduced me to the word "auspicate" years ago, and I've loved it ever since. According to Merriam-Webster, it's defined as:

1 *archaic:* to indicate in advance as though by an omen: PORTEND, AUGUR

2   to initiate or enter upon especially under circumstances or with a procedure (such as drinking a toast) calculated to ensure prosperity and good luck

To auspicate is to nurture and call in grace , to conjure an alignment with the benevolent forces of the universe, an incredibly pure, yet grounded, positive influence that we can apply to our lives—though it matters how we define and relate this intangible but-oh-so-real source of goodness.

What Is Luck, Really?

That's what luck really is—preparation meeting the moment of opportunity... You do the work. You do whatever is necessary to be prepared for whatever it is you're trying to acquire or attain or accomplish. And then you let it go. You release it. You release all attachment to the outcome, because you know you have done everything that you possibly can do. And when you've done everything you can do, that's the moment of surrender, release. And then if it's supposed to be yours, it will come to you.

—Oprah Winfrey[1]

This definition of luck captures the essence and meaning of auspicating. Preparing for the opportunity and doing everything we can to call in our desires is important because it tells the universe that we're ready. By doing the work, we create movement in our lives. That, in turn, catalyzes a response from the universe. The time, effort, and energy we contribute become a welcome mat that we lay down, so when grace does arrive, the atmosphere inside us and in our lives can support it.

While putting in the time, energy, and effort are nonnegotiables, pure, unfettered synchronicity also exists. Have you ever thought about someone you haven't seen in a long time, only to run into them out of the blue, in the unlikeliest of circumstances? Have you ever imagined an outcome and then watched in amazement as it came true before your eyes? This sort of magic happens, and it, too, is a form of grace, or synchronicity. Yet experienced this way, it unfolds without an obvious initial outlay of effort. We can, and often do, think and feel our desires into being. However, by putting in the work, by doing everything possible to prepare, we catalyze their arrival.

This idea harkens back to the "rose-colored realism" of resilient people we discussed in chapter 1. To practice rose-colored realism, we must be a realist *and* a consummate benefit finder: individuals who can find the benefit, and the meaning, of the stresses of life. This is the part where we show up and put in the time, the energy, the effort. Not because of an unrelenting work ethic but because of pure intention. As Oprah says, we do the work, and anything and everything we can to show up and prepare to receive. Once we've done that, if it's meant to be ours, we receive the benefits of grace.

Staying Committed to Grace

Grace, luck, and blessings all sound enchanting, but when we're busy living, navigating the inevitable twists and turns of our lives, we can sometimes forget to notice when, where, and how they show up. In especially hard times, we may also stop trusting that divine favor is real, or that grace exists at all. Instead, we may feel abandoned by the universe; this often happens during and after traumatic experiences, including loss and illness.

I've certainly felt cosmically forgotten in my own life. I wasn't born into affluence. My parents' contentious divorce created significant economic and emotional stress. Clinically depressed, I felt like my life was an unrelenting battle. Then, cancer knocked me down even harder. I didn't understand what menopause was when I had my hysterectomy as a teenager, let alone how to live with it for the rest of my life. My mental health became way worse with panic attacks and anxiety before it became better. Of course, I wanted to give up. Who wouldn't?

Because of my willingness to do the work, though, grace has always met me halfway. For years, I worked at my healing at every conceivable level, creating post-traumatic growth (PTG), which is positive change resulting from crisis or trauma. Coined by researchers Richard G. Tedeschi and Lawrence Calhoun, PTG is a possible outcome of post-traumatic stress disorder (PTSD).

Trusting in grace and showing up for the possibility of abundance in the face of loss and adversity is the ultimate act of resilience. It's the ability to bounce back, to *not* give up, to *not* stop trusting and believing in yourself and in life, especially when things get really tough. It's ultimately fueled by grit, the passion that rises from the soul to keep going. This same passion is precisely what commands circumstances to bow to your unrelenting desires for your life.

Positivity and Our Ever-Expanding Capacity

Cosmically, grace, positivity, luck, and blessings are all associated with the planet Jupiter, who also represents faith, hope, and optimism. In service to our highest good, he highlights our beliefs about life, including our personal philosophy.

The nature and essence of Jupiter are also firmly reflected in positive psychology. In fact, positivity — those feelings of contentment, joy, curiosity, and interest that we view as signs of well-being — has, in recent decades, become an important focus of research.

Barbara Fredrickson, renowned professor of psychology at the University of North Carolina at Chapel Hill, has spent much of her career researching positivity. Her resulting "broaden-and-build theory" tells us that positive emotions activate our brains to tune in to context and elevate our awareness, helping us to see the bigger picture.[2] Just like our friendly planet Jupiter, positive emotions expand our cognitive flexibility and creative capacities.

This resulting "broadened" state in turn promotes behaviors that help us build our physical, intellectual, and social resources. Curiosity facilitates learning and the integration of new knowledge. Play results in new and stronger social bonds. Contentment invites self-reflection and stronger self-knowing. In building these resources, we elevate our resilience and future capacities to cope in times of stress.

Compare this effect to what happens when we feel stricken with panic or anxiety. The only options we see in front of us are typically to fight or take flight. In that restricted mindset, we feel limited, oriented toward surviving rather than thriving, and in the process, we fail to seek the benefits of our circumstances.

The difference between what we do and don't notice in these two different states of mind is striking. Our feel-good emotions not only signal a current state of well-being but also produce greater health and expanded capacity. They literally help us better "resource" our future selves for more effective healing.

Elevating Our Positivity Frequency

I love the saying "My joy is my responsibility, and my responsibility is my joy," but what does it mean in the context of daily life? In the midst of turmoil, or even just a so-so boring day, being told to keep our "chin up" and "stay positive" feels insincere, if not downright grating. Yet also, there's a stark difference between engaging positivity for spiritual bypassing—i.e., playing at/faking "happy" to avoid doing the real work of digging in and cultivating true joy—and engaging positivity as a framework for resilience. Spiritual bypassing happens when we immediately jump to a positive feeling before processing pain, and usually, it is laced with denial.

The reality is, we need to stay disciplined with cultivating our happiness, just as much as we would commit to expanding any other character strength. Cultivating the positive, leaning into joy, noticing what's going well (as opposed to just highlighting what's going wrong), and understanding how even the worst circumstances might lead us to an expanded place of well-being in our lives—when adequately dealt with—can create resilience. There, in that place, we can bounce back from adversity stronger and find our way to grace, growth, and good fortune. By working on cultivating rose-colored realism as much as we can, we embrace the bounty of Jupiter and his countless gifts, which he willingly shares with us.

If you've read chapter 5 on the moon, you know that I'm an advocate for feeling all emotions. Recognizing the benefits of expression and compassion for all your feelings, even during dark nights of the soul, can provide you with a revolutionary breakthrough in emotional health. Don't forget feeling all of your emotions also means experiencing joy, hope, love, and pleasure. Engaging positivity, both by feeling it and by showing up to do the work to call in grace, in itself constitutes a radical choice on behalf of your cosmic health. Facing your toughest moments with a mindset of affirmation, acceptance, grit, and openness is an incredible act of courage and self-empowerment.

So how do we do this?

Practicing Positivity

Given that the primal brain was designed first and foremost to help us survive in ancient times, when we lived amidst tigers, bears, venomous snakes, and more, we're fundamentally programmed to detect danger. It's this part of the brain that initiates the fight-or-flight stress response. Since this tendency to emphasize the negative—which the primal brain perceives as threats to our survival—is so intertwined with our basic survival instinct, we have to work harder to balance out that bias toward the negative with exponentially higher degrees of positivity. In other words, we have to *decide* that we want to feel good, and then show up and do the work that allows those positive feelings and experiences to take shape inside us and in our lives.

These two realities are essential to calling in grace and the cosmic health it supports:

1. **We cannot expect to rid ourselves of negative affect.** Anxiety, sadness, and fear help us adapt and survive. They allow us to anticipate negative outcomes, prepare us to avert or manage risk, and then adjust to the outcomes. Anger, even rage, is sacred and imperative in order for us to protect, love, and honor ourselves and others. We need all of these emotions as well as our more positive ones. Emotions like fear aren't bad unto themselves. Without these survival-oriented emotions, we would never truly know the full extent and effects of positive affect. How could we possibly comprehend or appreciate joy, relief, or even laughter if we'd never known fear, regret, and anger?

2. *The more* **positivity we cultivate,** *the merrier* **we feel.** Literally, without negating or downplaying our challenging moments, we can enrich our health and our lives by cultivating and savoring moments of happiness. As a matter of fact, resilience is cultivated by acknowledging and processing hardship while also leaning into the positive. When we make an abiding commitment to positivity, we affirm the goodness of life. From that place we can access gratitude, joy, love, and hope, even if only in brief bursts. Like learning a new skill, cultivating positivity is a holistic daily practice that spans every layer of our being— body, mind, spirit, home, family, work, and so on.

Of course, the goal isn't to pressure ourselves to feel positive at all times, or at the drop of a hat. We want instead to consistently practice shifting our focus to the positive. It's a skill we need to cultivate consistently.

Numerous studies point to strategic ways we can prime ourselves for positive affect. Here are some approaches that have worked particularly well for me:

Practice gratitude. Recognize what you appreciate in the moment. If gratitude feels like a stretch, ask yourself: "What's going well?" See if you can conjure heartfelt appreciation, even if it's for the tiniest detail. A moment of thankfulness often inspires us to think creatively and abundantly, acting for the benefit of ourselves and others.[3]

Reframe the narrative. What would happen if you thought of your difficulty as a challenge to master, starring you as the hero? Recast yourself as the victor of the story, not the victim. Even if it doesn't feel plausible at first, it's important to retrain your brain to consider your power to change your story and your role in it. You can do this by writing or in conversation with someone you trust. This method of coping, called "positive reappraisal," is all about finding the nuggets of good within negativity. It particularly helps those in unimaginable circumstances of stress or loss.[4]

Be curious. Ask questions. Look around you. Consider alternative actions. Curiosity leads us to find novelty in the present moment. Not only do we learn more; we also activate mindfulness, which can support positive feelings.[5]

Choose empathy and compassion. When you embrace empathy and compassion as opposed to sympathy, you feel and display true loving-kindness. Sympathy, on the other hand, can seem insincere, even self-pitying. Empathy and compassion lead to feeling heard, understood, validated, and cared for, whereas sympathy can seem like a coping mechanism in the face of situations that you aren't adequately prepared for.[6]

Tackle your (realistic) to-dos. Whether you're faced with a seemingly insurmountable challenge or just a blah day, identifying and going after realistic goals can be the perfect remedy. When we chip away at those errands and make those decisions and plans—especially when they pertain to the painful point at hand — we regain a sense of efficacy and mastery over seemingly uncontrollable situations.[7]

Relentlessly commit to your future self. Crafting a vision of who you want to be in one, five, or twenty years compels you to make decisions that support your highest good. In doing so, you co-create a new reality with your future self.[8]

Notice that the focus is on action, not feeling. When we engage these actions, we create a mindset and environment that facilitates the flow of positive emotions. With consistency and commitment, we can regularly engage these practices, independent of how we currently feel. For me, this might look like going for a long walk, putting on headphones and blasting music, or taking micro-actions — packing a gym bag for tomorrow morning, or quickly handling an administrative task.

FEELING GOOD WHEN THINGS FEEL SHITTY

There's no denying that it can be hard to engage these practices amidst times of darkness. I've been there, in that place so wrought with difficulty that appreciation and gratitude, while present and available, don't give us enough juice to counter our negativity. This is when being grateful for the little things isn't sufficient to elevate our baseline emotional experience.

What do we do when gratitude isn't enough to realign our emotions with the positive, leaving us still stuck in a dark place?

I've found this four-step process enormously helpful, both for myself and my clients:

1. **Name what you're feeling and go into the specifics.** Take your attention into your body and locate what you're feeling. Is it a racing heart, tightening in your chest, clenching in your thighs? What does it feel like — butterflies, rapid pulsating,

throbbing pain? Name out loud where you feel the sensation(s) in your body and what it feels like. Keep your attention on the physical sensation(s) and notice how it shifts with your continued attention. Here's an example: "I feel restriction in my chest with a low, dull pain circulating around my heart, as if someone is pushing two hands into the core of my chest."

2. **Get clear on the emotion you're feeling.** Once you're clear on your physical experience, ask yourself what emotion is behind it. Is it grief, anger, jealousy? Don't censor yourself. Whatever it is, is okay. By claiming your disavowed feelings you can potentially liberate them. The key is figuring out what that emotion is asking you to acknowledge.

3. **Do something to discharge the energy in your body.** For me, this usually involves moving my body in a vigorous way, like taking a brisk walk, jumping up and down, or going jogging. However, back in the days when I was sick with cancer and rigorous physical activity wasn't an option, I opted for other forms of self-soothing, including rolling up into a ball and gently rocking back and forth. Even in smaller doses, movement allows the body to physically process and discharge energy. Consider what works for your body and choose a physical activity or action that feels comforting, even therapeutic. You can also release energy by yelling, doing chair yoga, or simple stretching.

4. **Breathe.** Connect with your breath and spend some time taking deep breaths with your eyes open. Anchor into your breath while simultaneously becoming present in the moment, including your immediate surroundings. Notice every sensory detail around you: the colors, scents, and sounds. What does the chair you are sitting in feel like? How about the floor you are standing on? Notice at least three details in your environment that stand out to you. Then continue to connect with your breath, taking air deeply into your abdomen, expanding your side rib cage, and continuing to

> breathe even more deeply into your upper rib cage and the
> clavicle region of your chest. When you exhale, release the
> clavicle region first, then the remainder of the upper rib cage,
> the side rib cage, and then the lower abdomen last. Repeat
> for at least four cycles.
>
> After you go through this four-step process, see if you can return
> your attention to the activities mentioned previously—gratitude,
> meaning, kindness, curiosity—to conjure some positivity.

Practicing More Ease and Grace

With consistent practice, this transition into a more positive state of mind gets easier and faster. The process happens in the reverse too: when we engage a mentality for broad thinking—by staying curious and being open to new possibilities—we invite more positivity into our minds and our lives. These effects are reciprocal; they accumulate and compound. This is what Barbara Fredrickson calls the "upward spiral."

Remember Mari, in chapter 2? As a bartender, she had gotten stuck in a super social, party-centric life of immediate gratification. Her goal of making a total life transformation, which in many ways sounded like a rags-to-riches, lonely-heart-to-true-love fairy tale, would have seemed like a pipe dream to many; the distance between where she was and the comparably luxurious life she wanted to conjure into existence was considerable. In spite of these seemingly steep odds, she worked really hard to hold on to hope, stay positive, and take consistent and definitive action toward her dreams.

Mari's vision was grandiose—as she always said of her dream life, "There will be champagne." In spite of the apparent distance between her service-industry life and her dream life, she continued to put herself, her health, and her spiritual transformation at the top of her priority list. By showing up again and again, she signaled to the universe that she was committed, and also ready to step into this new, more desirable version of her life. Now, as you may recall, she is happily married and living in a penthouse. She feels self-expressed, and as she once envisioned, there is indeed champagne when appropriate.

That's the power of setting intentions, showing up, doing everything possible to receive the abundance we desire. Whether in health, wealth, love, fulfillment, or any other areas, the most amazing transformations can and do happen when we show up and prepare to receive. By continually injecting ourselves with a spirit of hopefulness, optimism, energetic input, and upbeat commitment, we change at a deep and soulful level. In that place, we become cosmically healthy, able to conjure results we previously only imagined. It's an incredibly powerful place to be that sends a resounding "Yes!" to the universe as it steps out to meet us, doling out blessings from one day and one month to the next.

Connecting with Heartfelt Hope and Optimism

Jupiter is, without a doubt, one of my absolute all-time favorite planets. Far more than just a benefic planet delivering an ample dose of "good vibes," he is the ruler of Sagittarius and associated with religion, big-picture thinking, and long-distance travel. Sagittarius is a sign capable of blunt honesty, helping us to become really clear in matters of the heart and mind. As its ruler, Jupiter, too, can help us discover the clarity of mind and purpose that charts an entirely new and more elevated course for us and our lives. While my reasons for adoring Jupiter are manifold, among them are the ability to connect us with the parts of ourselves that long for adventure, spirituality, philosophy, and the true and lasting abundance that comes from expressing ourselves authentically.

Jupiter is a massive planet, boasting a diameter 11.2 times the size of Earth's (which, to keep things in perspective, is just 10 percent of the sun's diameter). This giant and almighty gift-giving planet encourages us to consider what makes a good life, connecting us to an understanding of our own belief systems and what we personally need for happiness and fulfillment.

Whenever Jupiterian astrological aspects are at play—whether it's Jupiter or Sagittarius—I encourage you to spend more time pondering your personal philosophy, the core concept that underlies why you do what you do and what you inherently believe to be true of life. This is a time to call in and cultivate something that informs who you are, how you live, and what you desire to create in this lifetime. This is a time to get out, go for it, and then, with Jupiter's help, bring it home.

Jupiter in Your Natal Chart: Putting It to Work for You

Where Jupiter shows up in your chart—which sign and house he was in at your time of birth—reveals where you naturally expand, have good luck, and are meant to shine. Jupiter reminds us of the necessity to feel good, have fun, lean into hope, and conjure creativity. A welcome planet, known to bring a "Go big" influence, Jupiter is the cosmic party guest you can't help but smile at.

As the largest planet in the solar system, Jupiter represents growth. Located five times farther from the sun than Earth, Jupiter takes twelve Earth years to orbit the sun. Visible from Earth with the naked eye, the planet was named by the Romans after the supreme god in Greek mythology, Zeus.

Jupiter transits that correlate positively to your personal chart also mark a time for opportunity. Jupiter encourages you to go for things that are bigger than you and more than you—especially if they expand you and the potential of your life. Focus outside yourself with a sense of devotion; significant achievements and breakthroughs *will* come.

Jupiter in Aries ♈: With Jupiter in this cardinal fire sign, you have a healthy sense of self-esteem, courage, and passion. Keeping a positive mindset helps you expand upon this natal blessing as does leaning into gratitude. Identify your strengths and leverage them. Manage your energy, not your time. Exercise helps you with this. You expand by inspiring and uplifting others, so don't hold back.

Jupiter in Taurus ♉: With Jupiter in this fixed earth sign, you are grounded, practical, and blessed with perseverance. You have a natural propensity toward the embodiment of pleasure. You are here to reclaim your connection to sensuality and model to others how to cultivate, nourish, and express this energy. Spending time in nature, nourishing yourself with delicious food, and making your body a comfortable place to be—via yoga, massage, stretching, and mindful movement—unlocks your luck.

Jupiter in Gemini ♊: With Jupiter in this mutable air sign, you are a mentally agile creative thinker who can be quite witty. Learning how to leverage your voice helps to unlock your luck. With Jupiter in Gemini, you have the capacity to write, communicate, and network with ease and power. You have a healthy sense of flexibility and can adapt to new or different situations. You cultivate ease by speaking your truth.

Jupiter in Cancer ♋: With Jupiter in this cardinal water sign, you excel at creating safety and security in your life by tending to your foundations: your primary relationships, your home, and your family. Emotionally you connect to others with your compassionate heart and empathetic understanding. While you excel in the role of the nurturer, you can also earn exceptionally well. Living in a home you love can help you to feel connected to your foundation.

Jupiter in Leo ♌: With Jupiter in this fixed fire sign, your creativity burns brightly. You are here to express yourself. Following your passion and doing what you love opens you up to greater joy, a higher vibration, and the ability to co-create your desires with ease. Staying in alignment with your values, your beliefs, and the parts of your life that hold the most meaning supports your success. When you are out of alignment with these aspects of yourself, life feels harder. Maintaining a confident and optimistic attitude creates opportunities for expansion.

Jupiter in Virgo ♍: With Jupiter in this mutable earth sign, the feel-good, positive influence of Jupiter combines with Virgo's integrity and practicality. You are adept at adhering to powerful practices around health, eco-consciousness, and other service-driven missions. For you, abundance looks like making a difference and staying focused on a concrete goal that betters the health of the world. Cultivating your service-driven nature is the key to unlocking your luck.

Jupiter in Libra ♎: As the feel-good, positive influence of Jupiter combines with the beauty and righteousness of this cardinal air sign, you can expect to excel at standing up for what you believe in, bonding deeply with a tight-knit community, adorning yourself stylishly, indulging your creative talents, and stepping more fully into a sense of empathy for others. Larger-than-life gains come from building community and pursuing service-driven missions, especially ones that create and support beauty, love, and justice.

Jupiter in Scorpio ♏: With Jupiter in Scorpio (fixed water), you are drawn toward intimacy. For you, unafraid of taboo topics, nothing is off the table. When you commit, you follow through with grace and determination. Exploring your sexuality and turning to orgasm is especially healing for you. Sensuality and pleasure allow you to experience the range of your existence and embrace your potential to co-create the biggest and brightest vision of your life.

Jupiter in Sagittarius ♐: Jupiter rules Sagittarius (mutable fire), so this placement showcases Jupiter in his dignity. You excel when you are aligned with your truth, your passion, and your most connected desires. Pursuing a personal philosophy that represents your core values remains paramount. When you lose your way in life, you can return again and again to your truth. Even though your truth will consistently shift and change as you grow, keeping your finger on the pulse of it remains nonnegotiable.

Jupiter in Capricorn ♑: With good-luck Jupiter in cardinal earth sign Capricorn, you excel at honoring your Saturn lesson and purpose. This placement can also highlight the role of stability. When you focus on the practicalities of your day-to-day without losing focus on your bigger picture, you shine. You are responsible and gifted with leadership and business. Your social consciousness may manifest through sustainable business practices and strong political views. Stay on the lookout for an obsessive need to succeed.

Jupiter in Aquarius ♒: With Jupiter in this fixed air sign, you crave freedom and the opportunity to be uniquely you. Tending toward all things eclectic, innovative, and intellectual, you excel at gathering groups of like-minded, wide-ranging people for a specific purpose — think rituals, politics, theater arts, mastermind groups. You seek out opportunities to mind meld in sometimes offbeat settings or in ways that venture just to, or even beyond, the bleeding edge.

Jupiter in Pisces ♓: With Jupiter in Pisces (mutable water), you expand when you turn to your emotions, imagination, and spirituality. Music, meditation, and the arts widen your periphery and help you hear deeply; this is how the mystical truths of the universe become available to you. You are likely no stranger to emotions, yet learning how to cry cathartically helps you purge what you no longer need. A steady and regular meditation practice is essential.

Jupiter in Retrograde

Since Jupiter is the astrological influence that expands, bestows gifts, and awakens our optimism, Jupiter's retrograde — which happens annually for approximately four months—is a time to look within and see where you're ignoring your intuition. Jupiter's retrograde is a time for your ego to reconcile where you're misaligned with the philosophies and truths that guide your life. However, if Jupiter is transiting retrograde in a part of your chart where he will touch a planet, it's an extra special time; it facilitates personal spiritual growth and possibly even financial growth. Jupiter's influence is notoriously good; however, he can also create the experience of "too much." So while he's in retrograde it's an opportune time to minimize and get back to basics. The key word for this retrograde is "truth."

Jupiter Ritual: Calling in Luck

This is a great ritual to do any time you want to connect with a higher vibration, or when Jupiter and the sun align, or around any new moon or full moon in Sagittarius, or near your birthday, or whenever you'd like to reignite your optimism and hope.

Before you begin working with Jupiter, look at your life, your home, your car, your email inbox, that stack of papers piled up on your desk, and the various other places in your life where metaphorical dust balls gather. Then ask yourself, *What am I avoiding in these areas of my life? And is there something in that mess that I need to handle?*

Co-creating luck requires that you cultivate your will and desire. As Oprah recommends, we do the work and prepare for grace to arrive. This means taking action on behalf of your dreams from a place of love, including getting the small things done—*no matter what.*

To begin this ritual, you will need one white candle, a pen, and a piece of paper. With these items nearby, sit at a table and journal on this question: *If everything in my life goes as well as it possibly could, what would happen?*

Freewrite your answer for twenty to thirty minutes, jotting down your dreams, visions, and ideas. Once you are finished, light your white candle. As you see the flame burning, know that you are igniting your passion and desire to live your absolute best life, and call in all the luck and magic that you can.

Review what you wrote and see what stands out. Take the written information and start to make a list of your most heartfelt desires. List as many as you'd like.

Once you're clear on what you want to call in, take a few moments to petition support from the universe. For some, this may look like prayer, and for others, a few moments of silence.

Next, ask yourself, *What can I start taking action on now?* Choose wisely. See where you can purposefully direct your intention and desire.

Notice what you are avoiding in your life. Big or small, make a plan to get it handled, like, now. Today. This week. For real. (The universe rewards immediate action.)

Make a plan to get one thing done each day that you've been putting off. This could be paying a bill, calling your mom, or returning that thing you borrowed from your friend but keep procrastinating on giving back. Whatever you've been procrastinating on, stop.

Schedule these tasks on your calendar, and no matter what, do them every day for an entire week.

With each difficult action you take, practice surrendering the outcome to the universe.

By moving through a whole week of accomplishing tasks, you are calling in Jupiter *and* creating the space in your life for opportunity to land.

CHAPTER 12

Saturn

Life Purpose and Discipline

About eight hundred miles south of Tokyo, Japan, is Okinawa Prefecture, an archipelago composed of 161 small islands. This region is home to the world's largest population of female centenarians. According to Dan Buettner, renowned longevity researcher and author of *The Blue Zones*, this is "ground zero for world longevity."[1]

In this part of the world, people enjoy the longest disability-free life on the planet. In addition to their physically active lifestyle, largely plant-based diet, modest food servings, and long-lasting social relationships, Okinawans live their lives with a deep sense of purpose, or *ikigai*.

Ikigai is often translated as "the reason for which you wake up in the morning." Okinawans believe that it's critical to have an enduring sense of purpose. Rather than suffering from disease and disability for years beforehand, Okinawans tend to die after a long, meaningful life, and also quickly, in their sleep. We see the positive ripple effects of healthy habits and *ikigai* in the 102-year-old martial arts master who is still actively teaching, and the 100-year-old fisherman who still fishes three times each week to feed his family.[2]

This same sense of purpose runs through other communities around

281

the globe where centenarians are more numerous and still living full, active lives. All of these communities, and the centenarians within them, adhere to their healthy lifestyles by relying on daily routines and fostering an abiding sense of community.

As we move forward in our journey toward cosmic health, next we'll explore the role of our habits and purpose in living our most vibrant and fulfilling lives. As appealing as that may sound, this is also the cosmic domain ruled by Saturn, whose heavy-handedness must not be overlooked.

An Abrupt, yet Necessary, Turn

From jovial, expansive Jupiter, we now turn to Saturn, a planet known for its no-nonsense structure and discipline. As the ruler of Capricorn, Saturn calls us to the mat with a focused, determined energy. While Saturn is often portrayed in purely negative terms — sometimes called a taskmaster, the lord of restriction, or the lord of karma — his role in our lives is both complex and monumental.

Saturn, which is associated with authority, places an emphasis on rules and hard lessons. Yet when we heed his wisdom and guidance, our health, well-being, and sense of purpose become more grounded. When we acknowledge and then acclimate to his unrelenting influence in our lives, we can bloom at a deep and soulful level. To get to this place and stay there, we must continually do the hard work that is demanded of us. We must exercise discipline and conscious determination to shun excess in favor of more useful and productive routines and habits. We must also be guided by his wisdom, not here and there or when crisis strikes but day after day, year after year, like clockwork.

In her powerful book *Saturn: A New Look at an Old Devil*, author Liz Greene compares Saturn to the beast-prince in *Beauty and the Beast*. Rather than presenting Saturn in purely negative terms, she provides a more thorough and enlightened understanding of Saturn's true nature, as well as his symbolic import in our lives and psyche:

Saturn symbolizes a psychic process as well as a quality or kind of experience. He is not merely a representative of pain, restriction, and discipline; he is also a symbol of the psychic process natural to all human beings, by which an individual may utilize the experiences of pain, restriction, and discipline as a means for greater consciousness and fulfilment.[3]

Greene then goes on to place Saturn in a more personal context:

Saturn is connected with the educational value of pain and with the difference between external values—those which we acquire from others—and the internal values—those which we have worked hard to discover within ourselves. Saturn's role as the Beast is a necessary aspect of his meaning, for as the fairytale tells us, it is only when the Beast is loved for his own sake that he can be freed from the spell and become the Prince.[4]

Saturn in Live Action

Saturn can show up in our lives in many different ways, but one example of Saturn's nature and influence is evident in Frank, my fitness trainer, whom I mentioned in chapter 10. He required that I commit to his regimen daily, and he was tough, bordering on unforgiving. However, he also knew what each of us in his program needed and what each individual body could handle. I sensed this about Frank, and I trusted him as a result. However, he consistently demanded far more energy and resilience than I felt I had to give. And each time, at his insistence and with his encouragement, I found myself achieving more than I'd previously thought I could.

Through the very real pain of Frank's workouts, I learned what it meant and how it felt to reinvest sweat and tears, time and energy, as well as effort and hope into a body, soul, and life that at a relatively young age had seemed to betray me. As the days turned into weeks, the more he pushed me, the more energized, confident, and grateful I felt. This is Saturn in a nutshell—a tough-love initiator calling us to apply ourselves and who delivers sweet gifts (sometimes sweeter than we imagined) when we follow through.

Saturn's power to re-create us and our lives by first highlighting where we need to grow and then not letting us off the hook when it comes to making necessary changes can feel like a relentless wrecking ball hitting us hardest where it hurts most. The idea that we must push ourselves beyond what seem to be our natural limits can be triggering. I get it, but this is what Saturn's work requires. He demands that we adhere to the lesson we need to master in order to realize our highest potential.

Eleven years ago, when I first had to give up gluten, I felt limited not just in my eating but also in my life. Suddenly I had to question food servers about ingredients. I had to examine menus before even thinking about eating out. Yet by now, the health benefits of being gluten-free for me are so numerous and so noticeable, it's become a nonnegotiable part of my life.

Even benefic Jupiter, who expands us and offers us a dose of positivity and good luck, can only expand us to the extent that we have "done" our Saturn—as in, heeded his call. While on the face of it, Jupiter and Saturn seem to have little in common, they're both about the rewards that come when we take responsibility, aim high, and buckle down in the moments that require more than we initially thought we had to give.

For all his force and foreboding, Saturn, in many ways, is our most powerful ally, our greatest champion—if and when we heed his demands and live our most productive and purposeful lives.

Saturn Return

You may have heard of the "Saturn return," a year during which Saturn returns to the zodiac sign it was in when you were born, which typically happens right around age twenty-eight to thirty. Like Mercury retrograde, mainstream society likes to frame this occurrence as one of the astrological bogeymen—a time of mayhem, upheaval, and dread.

With each planet, we can understand its transit in our personal natal chart according to its cycles. With Saturn's approximately twenty-nine-and-a-half-year orbit, we experience the cross-quarter milestones approximately every seven years (twenty-nine divided by four).

Consider how this maps to your life:

Age seven: Saturn's opening is square to your natal Saturn placement. You enter more formal schooling and a more independent period of childhood. You learn to read, do homework, do chores, and experience higher expectations from your parents and teachers.

Age fourteen: Saturn is opposite your natal Saturn placement. In your teenage years, a tough time for growth, you are tasked with individuating from your parents and often feel at odds with authority figures.

Age twenty-one: Saturn's closing is square to your natal Saturn placement. You enter an advanced season of responsibility. For some, this time is about graduating from college, starting a career, moving away from home, and supporting yourself financially, perhaps for the first time.

Age twenty-nine: Saturn returns to your natal Saturn placement. Saturn comes back to the zodiac sign at the time of your birth, asking you to revisit your Saturn lessons. This is often a significant turning point in your life.

Rachel, a Jewish woman living in Washington, DC, was a classic example of what can occur during a Saturn return. Running her own six-figure business, she was in a relationship with someone she was in love with but couldn't see herself with forever. At a time in her life when many of her friends were happily coupled, Rachel was feeling increasingly unsettled.

As we began working together, we initially looked at ways to grow her business, and with my coaching, she more than doubled her revenue. Soon, however, it became clear that money and success alone wouldn't make Rachel happy. With her natal moon in Scorpio, she has a deep yearning for more meaning and intimacy, and her relationship wasn't meeting her needs. Although positive in many ways, this particular relationship missed the mark when it came to building toward a mutually agreed-upon life vision.

Rachel also yearned to travel. She had a fierce need to grow, evolve, and explore. Her partner, however, was rigid and reticent about risk. Terrified to do what a Saturn return demands — eliminate something to make space to embody truth more deeply — she'd held on to her relationship even though she knew this person wasn't "the one" for her.

Using astrology, as well as mindfulness and positive psychology practices, we began to isolate her core blocks. As a double Virgo — Virgo sun and rising — Rachel is adept at refining things down to their purest essence to create more order. She dreaded the challenging emotions that would arise if she ended her relationship. She feared that they would be so messy she'd be unable to live through the chaos they'd create. That fear had also been validated by her pattern of emotional eating, a coping mechanism that left her feeling even less capable of managing her big emotions.

The pressure of her Saturn return did eventually help Rachel end her relationship. The breakup was heart-wrenching and overwhelming at first, but it also gave her a new reason to move toward her deep desire for intimacy, meaning, and, someday, a family of her own. Several months later, Rachel took off with a backpack, heading to New Zealand on a solo travel adventure. She traveled, alone, for three months. A year after returning, she met her match. They have since married and are building a life based on mutual values.

Saturn return can manifest in any number of ways, but most often it's a time when we are cosmically tested, asked to revisit lessons we've learned (and those we've not yet learned). We are asked to commit to our highest good by choosing the right path, even when it's not the easiest one. This is a powerful time when we can align with our soul and apply our blood, sweat, and tears by making the necessary sacrifices and substitutions to create a daily life that's in sync with our *ikigai.*

To meet these challenges, we often have to reexamine how we're tending to our health (*Do I have the necessary habits in place to support lasting well-being, inside and out?*). We also may be asked to look at our daily schedule (*Am I living rhythmically, and if not, what needs to change?*) and whether we say no to people, activities, and obligations that don't serve our purpose (*Am I putting enough of my energy into realizing my potential?*).

Saturn, and Saturn return in particular, doesn't hesitate to bring hard decisions and seemingly insurmountable challenges to our door. In fact, when that's what's needed, Saturn knows it, and like Frank, he'll push us to run those extra miles we're not sure we can run...until somehow, in spite of all odds, we do exactly that.

Defining "Purpose"

The idea of purpose not only is embedded in Saturn's realm. It is also subjective, alluring, and at times overwhelming, even frustrating. For all its grandeur and aspiration, many find it hard to pin down a definition. When asked, "What is your purpose in life?" we tend to pause.

In my own work, I have come to define "purpose" as a commitment to a vision that motivates me. I view my purpose from both a long-term and a short-term lens, and base it on the values that matter most to me.

Your sense of purpose should be uniquely yours. It should reflect who you are, what you value, and how you intend to contribute to the world. To be sufficiently motivating, your purpose should carry deeply inspiring personal significance. Here are some questions to ask yourself as you craft your purpose statement:

What group or cause do I dream of serving?
What kinds of activities do I do willingly, even when they require hard work and dedication?

Why do I enjoy these activities or pursuits?

Who was I as a child, and what did I love doing then?

Start noticing these propensities, and journal about them when you do. Even if you already have purpose in your life, becoming consciously aware of it can help you to cultivate even more, and in so doing, elevate your cosmic health further!

Whatever your purpose, research shows that what matters is not what your purpose is but that you have one in the first place. Those who have a deep sense of purpose experience lower stress levels and decreased mortality compared to peers who do not possess a strong life purpose.[5] Researchers have found this to be true regardless of socioeconomic status, race, gender, or education level. In fact, the results of these studies suggest that adopting a sense of purpose is more powerful in decreasing the risk of death than abstaining from drinking and smoking, or even exercising regularly.

Whoa.

As surprising as that may seem, this finding makes a lot of sense. Why would anyone take any action toward sustained health, well-being, and making a contribution to the world if they didn't believe any of it would matter in the end? Purposefulness is a basic psychological need; it acts as a source of clarity, drive, and self-worth.[6]

When we connect with purpose, we are less likely to let the little things stress us out, anger us, or otherwise negatively control our lives. We are more likely to engage effective coping strategies as well. Think about it: if you sincerely believe that your life matters, you are all the more likely to take good care of yourself. In fact, having a higher sense of purpose is linked with increased movement, greater use of preventive health services, and less time in the hospital.[7]

A sense of purpose is associated with "eudaemonia," a concept that dates back to Aristotle and even earlier, to Socrates and Plato. Present-day scholars define eudaemonia as follows:

[W]ell-being is not so much an outcome or end state as it is a process of fulfilling or realizing one's daimon or true nature—that is, of fulfilling one's virtuous potentials and living as one was inherently intended to live.[8]

Eudaemonia comes from an all-encompassing well-being—living a life of meaning and self-actualization—as opposed to hedonic well-being, which focuses on pleasure seeking and pain avoidance. Yes, living in alignment with your purpose brings self-satisfaction and contentment, but it typically also necessitates hard work and, at times, distress, even sacrifice. In true Saturnian form, purpose-driven, or eudaemonic, living teaches us that some of the greatest rewards come through commitment to demanding yet worthwhile ideals.

Living (and Redefining) a Meaningful Life

Understanding your purpose is a lifelong pursuit, and a beautiful one at that. Personally, I have found that witnessing new iterations of my purpose unveil themselves is a joy in itself.

Instead of putting pressure on yourself to declare your ultimate and final purpose in life, see it as a path of discovery—one you can explore with each twist in your life, as well as each shift in the planet's cycles.

Living a purpose-driven life is so valuable in part because it infuses your daily life with enduring meaning, though let's be honest: sometimes it involves some drudgery. Researchers Frank Martela and Michael F. Steger identified three distinct aspects that, when combined, inform meaning in life:

1. **Coherence (or making sense of the world):** This speaks to our cognitive need to understand the wholeness of our lives and establish a sense of predictability. Interestingly, astrology provides us with that very sense of coherence by helping us better

understand ourselves and our lives. Remember the cosmic curriculum — how each of our natal charts illuminates our path and the lessons we must learn along the way to self-actualization? When we start to understand our natal chart in more depth, we develop coherence in our comprehension of who we are. When we start to understand the cycles of the seasons that guide our life, we increase coherence and, in the process, amplify our ability to develop meaning in our life.

2. **Purpose (in the form of goals and a sense of direction for the future):** As we've discussed, feeling aligned with our unique sense of purpose can improve our health and extend our life span. Purpose motivates behaviors, boosts self-esteem, provides perspective, and allows us to ride the waves of life.

3. **Significance (in terms of assessing the value and importance of life from a past, present, and future perspective):** By living with purpose, we are more likely to have an impact — to feel like our life matters. Knowing that we matter makes purpose worthwhile; it gives us a reason to work through the hard times — because who we are and what we do make a difference. Ultimately, this means reinforcing our belief that we matter because we exist. Remember, we share some of the same basic elements of burnt-out stars. We are intimately connected to the universe.

Granted, in this framework, purpose is just one of the three facets of a meaningful life, but Martela and Steger also underscore the interconnectedness of these three elements. It is difficult for one to exist without the others.[9] Without a sense of coherence, we would not be able to identify worthwhile goals that contribute to a purpose, and without significance, our purpose would likely lose its meaning. This exploration of meaning overlaps with what Liz Greene so expertly defines as a "fundamental psychological need for rhythm and ritual, the careful ordering of . . . inner life."[10]

Connect with Your Purpose

1. **Know your natal Saturn.** What element is your Saturn in? Is it water, earth, air, or fire? What is the lesson of that element for you? Refer to Saturn's position in your natal chart for more detail.
2. **Start a conversation.** Talk to people you know well and trust deeply. Ask them how they see you, what you do for them and others, what they feel you bring to the proverbial table of life.
3. **Write your own eulogy.** How would you like people to remember you and your life? Take a little time to write out how you'd like to be eulogized.
4. **Don't wait. Build.** Build meaning into your life. Do things that feel worthwhile. Cultivate your passions and hone skills that feel important to you. Spend your time wisely, with the goal of gaining more meaning and purpose in your life.

Remember, there are many ways to live your purpose throughout the different stages of life. If you find profound meaning in nurturing children, you may feel fulfilled in your working years as a preschool teacher and then find empowerment in your purpose by volunteering at a library or taking care of your grandchildren in your later years. Beware of tying your life's meaning to a specific job, role, or pursuit, or any sole iteration of your purpose. In a comprehensive study of longevity, researchers found higher rates of mortality in one's first year of retirement, suggesting that a loss of a sense of purpose can derail our health in the most serious of ways.[11] You are not worthy because you do. You are worthy because you are.

Committing to Your Purpose, Saturn Style

Saturn demands determination and hard work. He asks that you show up consistently for the habits and routines that create meaning in your life. I can't say this enough: Saturn is not something you pay attention to only at your Saturn return or when crisis strikes. He requires your daily attention. He is ultimately here to support you but never to enable or entitle you. His rewards are considerable, but they only come after you show up and do your full part.

Saturn in Your Natal Chart: Putting It to Work for You

Saturn's stern influence on our lives is undeniable, yet as we've seen, it exists to help us fulfill our potential and live meaningful lives. In Liz Greene's words: "it is through him alone that we may achieve eventual freedom through self-understanding."[12]

As the cosmic embodiment of tough love, Saturn forces us to live with integrity by upholding the health and work habits necessary to support a meaningful life. Saturn fulfills his own role by doing everything he can to prevent us from living inauthentic lives. He wants us to self-actualize at the highest level, and he's willing to push us further than we think we can go—which, again, is his way of teaching us what to do and what to avoid—to reorient our lives toward a more intentional direction. He has our back in the most profound of ways, and he's not afraid to rattle us at our very core when that's what's needed. Even so, his lessons often come through painful circumstances, which is why he has such a tough reputation.

Here's how Saturn can play out in your life, based on your natal chart placement:

Saturn in Aries ♈: With Saturn in Aries (cardinal fire) you are here to learn how to experience the freedom of being yourself. While this task comes with significant challenges, with consistent effort, determination, and personal responsibility, you are primed to achieve personal sovereignty. I know, asserting yourself feels scary, but asking for what you need, prioritizing your desires, and holding your boundaries prevents resentment.

Along similar lines, learning how to feel, honor, and express your anger in healthy ways is a critical part of your life lesson.

Saturn in Taurus ♉: With Saturn in Taurus (fixed earth), leaning into pleasure and learning how to trust your body offers you the pathway to liberation. Developing practices for self-nurturing and deep, soul-driven self-care expands your capacity to nourish others. While you may feel obliged to stay loyal to patterns of society, culture, and family, you are also here to flip the patriarchy upside down. That's easier said than done, yet by harnessing your relentless commitment, fierce determination, and grit, literally anything is possible.

Saturn in Gemini ♊: Saturn in Gemini (mutable air) asks you to master your mindset and your communication skills. With your insatiable thirst for learning, you may always be on a quest to know more, and maybe also to "prove" your knowledge and wisdom. Even in social settings where there's a need to belong, you may feel intimidated or hold back from networking. Regardless, you are here to bridge communities, expand networks, and facilitate the dissemination of knowledge, especially your most sacred and holy knowledge.

Saturn in Cancer ♋: With Saturn in Cancer (cardinal water), prioritizing emotional self-care is especially important. Finding reciprocity with how you give and receive emotional support with others remains key to your well-being. Consider your relationship with your mother and the matrilineal line in your family. What patterns are you here to disrupt, transform, or overcome? What are the qualities of your mother and her lineage that you want to preserve and develop?

Saturn in Leo ♌: With Saturn in Leo (fixed fire), your fear of self-expression may, at times, feel larger than life. Yet you are here to learn self-expression, self-discipline, and courage. Consider your relationship with your father. Pinpointing how you were or weren't nourished paternally can offer clues about what you need to forgive and integrate on your path to creative expression, personal sovereignty, and living a life of authentic expression. Spoiler alert: you are meant for all of this, yet it may be painfully difficult to express your full range of uniqueness.

Saturn in Virgo ♍: Shakespeare's "To thine own self be true" is the rallying cry for Saturn in Virgo (mutable earth). Yet learning to trust yourself, rather than berate yourself, can be challenging with this placement. With effort, you can achieve this. You are here as a leader who supports others. To support your health, Saturn asks that you integrate and deepen your mind–body–spirit connection, which forms the holy trinity of well-being. Developing a sincere focus or purpose for your life also helps you immensely.

Saturn in Libra ♎: With the disciplinarian of the sky in Libra (cardinal air), the sign of the scales, your life lesson centers around justice and developing an equanimous mind. That means accepting, and even welcoming, both "good" and "bad" experiences with equal fervor, knowing that you can leverage both. While your objectivity can sometimes be misunderstood as timid, your fair-minded nature doesn't lack conviction. You simply strive for balance no matter what. Accepting life's fluctuations allows for a peaceful inner existence. You, however, need to be mindful of codependent dynamics. Learn how to be in relationships with others.

Saturn in Scorpio ♏: With Saturn in Scorpio (fixed water), the sign of transformation, you go deep. You're meant to transcend the superficial and penetrate the unsaid. While this can be challenging, consider how much of life is spent denying the raw truth of what's going on. You have a knack for seeing into and beyond the shadows, secrets, and shame, looking straight into the heart of truth. Your sexuality remains incredibly important to your health and well-being. Learning what turns you on is nonnegotiable. You are unrelenting, and this serves you well, so long as you value your grit, tenacity, and personal strength. Self-love and self-acceptance are at the heart of your cosmic curriculum.

Saturn in Sagittarius ♐: With Saturn in Sagittarius (mutable fire), your life lesson revolves around faith. Learning to trust the essential goodness of the universe and developing faith in yourself remains crucial to your spiritual development and the ownership of your life purpose. While this placement might feel a bit depressive, staying aligned with hope and committed to your highest potential is worth the effort. When you do the work, your innate propensity for thought leadership shines brightly. You are a teacher. Don't be afraid to tell it like it is and offer your wisdom to the world.

Saturn in Capricorn ♑: Saturn in Capricorn (cardinal earth) brings matter-of-fact, nose-to-the-grindstone tendencies. Saturn rules Capricorn, so having Saturn in his sign of dignity in your natal chart means that responsibility comes naturally to you. Achievement, honor, and ambition are a big focus. Yet more importantly, doing the work to honor your own authority and peace of mind reflects the true essence of this Saturn placement. Learning how to bend, but not break, is crucial, as is the art of doing nothing (easier said than done). Be mindful of work addiction but understand that you are here to lead.

Saturn in Aquarius ♒: With Saturn in Aquarius (fixed air), learning to accept your common humanity remains paramount to your healing. Saturn is one of Aquarius's co-rulers, so Saturn in this placement has a natural aptitude. Yet given Aquarius's focus on being evolutionary and progressive, Saturn in this sign can have you feeling a persistent need to do better, be more, and have a greater impact. Saturn in this sign also asks for a commitment to the advancement of society. Learning how to accept yourself, not because you "do" but because you are, remains key for this Saturn placement.

Saturn in Pisces ♓: With Saturn in Pisces (mutable water), you have a distinct purpose in this life: to embody your spirituality. Yet that path is potentially laced with martyrdom and wondering *Why me?* If that's the case, learning self-compassion goes a very long way, as does the power of a good reframe. Inherently, we are all connected. You get that in your soul. Your life is about service, art, spirituality, compassion, and growth. Develop your boundaries, learn to say no, and no matter what, trust your intuition. Turn to music and art as much as you need to. They help you to unlock your healing magic.

Saturn in Retrograde

Retrogrades often bring a change in perspective, which can be disorienting at first. When Saturn goes retrograde, which he does annually for about four-and-a-half months, we feel the weight of our responsibilities. We may also feel temporarily disconnected from our purpose, and therefore less motivated to tend to those responsibilities. Saturnian aspects, including tradition, structure, rules, and foundations, may all be affected or need to be reassessed during Saturn retrograde.

Unlike some other planets, Saturn essence can become stronger, rather than weaker, when in retrograde position. As a result, his ability to put boundaries in our way is enhanced during his yearly retrograde. As harsh as this can sometimes feel, remember that Saturn pushes us to our limits, *not* beyond them. He wields his power when he must, and because we have not previously heeded his calls or warnings. On the flip side, however, Saturn retrograde can be a time of deep learning, a powerful time to revisit and readjust our routines, structures, habits, and purpose.

Saturn is among our toughest teachers, yes, but he's also our most faithful guide. When he's in retrograde, he's fulfilling this role by asking us to look back at the ground we've already covered and, when necessary, retrace our steps to redo or revise our plans so that we can move ahead in a more steady and grounded way once he turns direct.

Saturn Ritual: Finding Your Purpose

This is a ritual that will support you whenever you're ready to make a commitment to your transformation, regardless of the astrological alignments.

First take time to think about moments in your life when you felt engaged, absorbed, and excited by what you were doing. What was happening that helped you feel connected to a purpose?

Now think about the future you most desire to live. What about this vision most excites you? Begin to draw conclusions about your highest-level commitments and your deepest values.

- *What am I here to do?*
- *What's driving my life?*
- *What are my unique gifts, talents, and strengths?*

Use the questions I posed on pages 287–288 as a guide to craft your purpose statement. Doing this could take a few minutes, hours, or days, but don't let it extend longer than a week. Commit to exactly what your purpose is now. You can always change it later.

Once your purpose statement is written, it's time to have a commitment ceremony.

Take your purpose statement and read it out loud to yourself in front of the mirror three times. Take a moment to look yourself straight in the eye and listen to what's happening inside your head. Is there talkback? Doubt? Listen to your thoughts.

Then, once again, look yourself in the eye and affirm your intention by repeating it aloud three more times. Sit down and fold your paper with your purpose statement on it three times. With each fold see yourself stepping into this purpose. Once it's folded, draw Saturn's glyph (see page 51) on top. As you are drawing the glyph, see yourself accepting the support of Saturn to stay disciplined and structured as you create your future.

CHAPTER 13

Chiron

Why Your Wound Is Your Wisdom

Chiron, the "wounded healer," comes to remind us of the value of our deepest, most searing emotional and physical pain points. While he cannot erase the wounds themselves, he does show us the wisdom we have gained from them and how it can be channeled toward healing.

Next, we'll consider the value of looking inward, reconciling with our deepest pain, and, from that place, emerging as the wounded yet powerful healers that we, like Chiron, are here to become.

Viewing Wounds as Guiding Lights

Wounds show up in different forms. There may be a clear past trauma that we pinpoint as a root of ongoing difficulty. Or a core wound may be just as deep-seated yet without a clear point of origin. No matter the form, and despite the creeping anguish that we struggle to shake off, our suffering is never in vain.

Here are *some* of the core wounds that can haunt us, even decades after they occur.

- Trauma
- Body image issues
- Deep-seated insecurity or feelings of inadequacy
- Feelings of instability
- Fear of rejection
- Low confidence or sense of self-worth
- Addiction
- Feelings of blame or resentment
- Shame
- An unresolved feeling about a particular area of our life
- Perceived imperfections that nag at us
- A strained or nonexistent relationship with a parent
- Being orphaned, literally or metaphorically
- Cultural wounding; feeling othered by society

Does any of this ring a bell? I know it does for me. Our core wounding feels like the recurring antagonist in our story. Just when we think everything is amazing, there the villain appears again, reminding us that the struggle continues. This emotional albatross feels like the bane of our existence, the hole we can't seem to fill, the thing—no matter how much therapy we do—that we can't seem to move beyond, erase, or undo.

Yet what Chiron asks of us is to take a different perspective altogether. This vulnerability, while overwhelming, does not have to thwart us. We can learn to leverage our wounds—not erase them or require their resolution but rather coexist with them. We can develop compassion for them and because of them.

With patience, kindness, and understanding, we can ultimately view our wounds as our most powerful teachers, and therefore as some of our most valuable assets. When we face our pain, we can learn from it and become more evolved versions of ourselves. Integrating the lessons of Chiron is about sitting with our hurts and accepting that they may never fully go away. In so doing, we continually remind ourselves that we can survive, even thrive, with the emotional scars that remain inside us.

Chiron is ultimately a celestial influence of empathy and compassion; his essence in our chart illuminates the darkness that gives way to dawn.

Healing from Wounds Written in the Stars

Chiron points to a sensitivity that represents immense potential for growth. This is a lifelong process, and anything even remotely resembling sorrow can trigger anguish. In these moments, the mind and body might cope by trying to run away or avoid these triggers. Ultimately, however, this experiential avoidance runs counter to our well-being.[1]

Conversely, we may rub salt into the wound since we are biologically programmed to wallow in painful memories. This is evolution's way of helping us remember the tough lessons we've learned so we don't repeat them. Unfortunately, this tendency toward intrusive rumination reinforces the brain's pathways for suffering. If left unchecked, the way we talk and think about our vulnerabilities may cause us to continually relive our traumas. Martha Beck, bestselling author and renowned life coach, explains the benefits and perils of our emotional healing process this way:

> Humans also have a unique way of recovering from trauma: We need to share our hurts. Fortunately, pretty much everyone now knows that talking to a compassionate, nonjudgmental person can heal emotional wounds. But when our cultural focus on "the talking cure" joins forces with our natural inclination toward negativity, we can get stuck.[2]

The process of healing, then, seems like a catch-22. We are the products of our history, a composite of the universe and of the past we have lived. Much of our healing requires us to look back in order to make wise choices for the future. But how do we do so if that is just going to reactivate our pain?

The key is to acknowledge and act on pain in a way that facilitates growth and healing, to learn how to feel our feelings without becoming our feelings. That ultimately means observing and witnessing feelings without further investing in them as our identity. The more willing we are to name and handle our wounds, the more likely we are to create harmony within our lives.

Spirituality, Pain, and Healing

Standing in front of the de Young Museum in San Francisco's Golden Gate Park, I could feel the waves of grief and sadness rippling through me, tearing at my insides and turning me into a walking, talking hub of waterworks. I would never be able to have kids, and adoption was seeming increasingly unlikely. My deep yearning to become a mother would be left unmet forever.

As I explained what was happening to my friend, whom I had flown to visit, she looked concerned but also confused. With utter sincerity, she turned toward me and said, "I don't understand. You're a spiritual person, and you believe that things happen for a reason. So why do you feel so much pain?"

The question jarred me briefly in that moment, but it also initiated an important discussion about spirituality and pain that falls squarely in Chiron's domain.

First, to be clear, we *can* be spiritually "positive" and grieve at the same time. Like cosmic health, we too embody the "both/and"—a duality, even a multiplicity, that allows us to be and feel several different traits, ways of being, and emotional states at once.

For the record, I also don't believe that everything happens for a reason. Nor do I believe that we "manifest" illness. The fact is, we are human and vulnerable to illness. We get sick or suffer deep pain for any number of legitimate reasons. We may have a predisposition. We may experience an unavoidable misfortune or trauma. We go through things—that's life!

As a spiritual person, I do believe that we can find a reason for everything that happens, that we can choose to unearth new levels of wisdom, forgiveness, and compassion as a result of pain, hardship, and heartache. We can decide to view our pain as our most powerful and relevant teacher. Being spiritual does not insulate us from pain or preclude us from experiencing it. Faith can, however, transform how we relate to our pain. When we accept our own multifaceted nature, we also accept that it's normal, even healthy, to suffer and heal simultaneously. As my mentor Dr. Maria Sirois always said, we can be broken and whole at the same time.

When I explained this to my friend in the middle of Golden Gate Park, she understood. The truth was, I'd known from a young age that I wouldn't have kids of my own. It came to me as a psychic premonition. When I learned I needed a hysterectomy at age nineteen, I felt "prepared" for the fact that I wouldn't have children. However, entering menopause at such a young age proved to be emotionally, psychologically, and physically grueling. When I reached my thirties, the grief of not being able to have children hit me like a tsunami.

While I can never reverse this fact about my body or my life, I eventually realized that I could use this torment as a way to understand the difficulties of others. In my toughest moments after my cancer, when my world felt annihilated, in the depths of despair, I'd repeat my mantra "None of this is in vain." I knew I'd take my experiences, as grueling as they felt, and support others who similarly suffered. This was Chiron acting as my teacher. You, like Chiron, are meant to do the same.

Healing through Self-Compassion

Self-esteem has long been considered the holy grail of psychological health, the key to true and lasting emotional well-being. I believe it was 2013 when I first heard Dr. Kristin Neff, a self-compassion researcher and associate professor at the University of Texas at Austin, present her revolutionary, arguably antiestablishment, perspective on self-esteem.

According to Dr. Neff's research, self-esteem has caused us some harm, partly because it's based on comparing ourselves to others. This tendency has contributed to an excessive focus on appearance and achievement. As a result, our quest for self-esteem could ultimately lower our self-worth, rather than raise and reinforce it.

Our focus instead should be on self-compassion, which her research has shown to be as empowering and motivating as self-esteem but without its pitfalls. When we have compassion for ourselves, self-soothing lowers our stress and enables us to be more present in the moment, allowing us to perform at higher levels.[3]

This emphasis on self-compassion is especially helpful when we're integrating our Chiron lesson. Rather than holding ourselves to impossibly perfect standards, we can treat ourselves as we do our friends and loved ones — with support, kindness, and encouragement. It's a radical idea, really, since we tend to feel justified in saying mean things to ourselves that, as Dr. Neff points out, we wouldn't ever say to someone we care about, or even to someone we don't like.

Have you ever noticed that? We tend to meet our own pain and challenges with pessimism, sometimes even rageful thoughts. Yet when our friends come to us for support, often with challenges that parallel our own, we rise to the occasion and provide loving care.

As Nitika Chopra, chronic illness advocate and founder of Chronicon, says, "Self-love means being more committed to your happiness than your suffering, in every moment."[4] That's a beautiful way to bottom-line the power of mindful self-compassion.

Self-Awareness and Mindful Self-Compassion

There are practices we can use to cultivate self-compassion. When I use them with clients, the difference is striking. Rather than indulging in exaggerated self-pity parties and negative self-talk, they begin to see themselves with self-understanding and love. By disengaging from thought processes that activate the fight-or-flight stress response, they begin to experience the "broadened" sense of positivity we learned about in chapter 11. This supports feelings of safety and security that help them to co-create new levels of cosmic health and well-being.

The building blocks of self-compassion are:

1. **Be with your emotions.** Notice your emotions and your experience. Practice validating them to yourself, acknowledging that what you are going through may be difficult, but it is also human. Remember Rachel from the Saturn chapter who during her Saturn return had to learn how to be with difficult, intense emotions? Her growth lay in her ability to be present with her emotions when they showed up in her body. By doing so, she made important changes that ultimately transformed her health and her life.

2. **Comfort and protect.** Soothe yourself in times of distress. Sometimes it's helpful to start by focusing on what's happening in your body. This may mean noticing the tightness in your chest, the churning in your belly, the clenching in your jaw. Whatever you experience in response to stress, take a moment to notice it. This helps to refocus your mind on experiencing greater self-compassion, which brings feelings of calm and safety.

3. **Provide for your needs.** Often we know what we need but feel unable or unwilling to get it. At this stage, it's often helpful to envision a wise, trusted acquaintance. This may be a friend, a parent, a longtime doctor or specialist. What would they "prescribe" if they met you in this moment? What would it tangibly look like to stay more committed to your happiness than to your suffering?

Self-compassion orients us to a life of resilience, health, and well-being. When we treat ourselves like we do our friends and loved ones, we begin to make choices that align with our long-term goals and vision, rather than satisfying the short-term gratification that too often sabotages our overall health and happiness. To learn more go to centerformsc.org.

Another Opportunity for Post-Traumatic Growth

Our capacity to heal is far greater than we imagine. If you live with a chronic illness or painful circumstances that are beyond your control, you may doubt this. With my own diagnosis, there was a time when I thought I was doomed, that I could not possibly live a life in pursuit of my goals while also fighting for my health. Healing takes many forms, and while, no, I could not individually remove every cancerous cell from my body or magically reimplant ovaries inside me, I eventually started looking at what I could do, in the open space of my new reality — even after being catapulted into menopause in my teen years, and even without motherhood in my future.

The essence of post-traumatic growth is achieving a life that is better than it was before. From this perspective, trauma and misfortune become a doorway to positive change. Those who enter into post-traumatic growth (a concept introduced in chapter 11) reap the benefits of a renewed appreciation of life and stronger relationships with others. The experience of pain brings them greater knowledge of their strengths and capabilities and leads them toward new purpose-driven goals with a reinvigorated life-philosophy.

By practicing mindful self-compassion, and moving through difficulty with acceptance and productive hopefulness, we guide our recovery in a transformative way, beyond "fixing" what was "broken."

Chiron's Story: Healing Others in Spite of His Pain

The myth of Chiron shows us our healing power often stems from the pain we endure. A centaur — half man, half horse — Chiron should have been as wild and vulgar as his fellow centaurs. Known for living without law and order, centaurs stormed fields and trampled crops. The centaurs' young were often spanked, kicked, and left to fend for themselves. Not surprisingly, they then grew up to be as lawless as their parents.

Chiron was an exception among his fellow centaurs. Known for his kindness and wisdom, he was warm, loving, and wise, especially to children. While he appeared to be related to other centaurs, in fact he was the immortal son of Cronus the Titan (Saturn is the Roman variant of Cronus) and notably different in disposition.

Due to his talents as a healer, Chiron became known as the greatest teacher in Greece. In his serene cave on Mount Pelion, Chiron schooled his students in sports, how to use healing herbs, and how to read the stars. He famously taught Achilles.

Yet Chiron was wounded at an early age. His mother, Philyra, a nymph, abandoned him when she birthed him, out of shock—she didn't know that she was pregnant with a centaur. His father's rendezvous with Philyra had been one of deceit, so he also denied his son's existence. As an orphan, Chiron lived his life with the hurt of his parents' rejection. Apollo, however, took him under his wing, nurturing him and his talents into existence.

Sadly, Chiron was destined for another pain. One day his friend Hercules accidentally struck his leg with a poisonous arrow, which should have killed him, but because he was Cronus's son, he was immortal and couldn't die. Instead of succumbing to the arrow injury, Chiron lived with physical pain, which only compounded his original childhood warning.

Chiron's story teaches us that we can endure great pain and use it to animate our capacity to empathetically relate to, and even heal, others. It also shows us that while a wound itself—a trauma or an emotional scarring—may never be erased, we can leverage the pain it has caused, and become wiser and more compassionate as a result. Our wound, then, offers us a path to personal mastery, potentially even serving as a source of wisdom to help others to heal.[5]

Chiron Return

"Centaur" is a term used not just for a mix of man and horse but also for a celestial body that resembles both a comet and an asteroid. Flying between the courses of Saturn and Uranus, Chiron follows an erratic fifty-year orbit. (Because of Chiron's placement between Saturn, the last of the ancient planets, and Uranus, many consider Chiron to be the spiritual key that unlocks the consciousness of the outer planets.)[6]

Due to his central role in our emotional healing and evolution, Chiron's lessons revisit us in significant ways via the Chiron return, which occurs close to our fiftieth birthday. This is often a time of realization, a turning point at which we revisit our Chiron wound and learn to integrate its lessons in deeper and more powerful ways.

When we commit to our Chiron work and are willing to show up wholeheartedly for the healing process it can provide us, Chiron return can liberate our potential—again, not in spite of our core wound but because of it.

We see this in Chiron's own story. After enduring the physical wound, he offered to change places with Prometheus, who was imprisoned for stealing fire from the gods to liberate humanity. In so doing, he became the ultimate healer, willing to sacrifice his physical being to relieve another's suffering.

For many, Chiron return offers a similar opportunity—to shift priorities and unleash our healing potential. It asks us who we are and what we want to do and be throughout our next phase of life. As Brian Clark, astrologer, explains:

> Hopefully what chooses to die are the misshapen and inauthentic parts of self. The initiation could then help reorder priorities, relinquish what is no longer appropriate or authentic and liberate the unlived spirit...In reality, the spirit is often chained up in the cellar, buried under ancestral rubble, until the wound of living has reached its density then spirit bursts through.[7]

Around the time of her Chiron return, a client of mine named Isobel, a white, queer artist living in Vancouver, experienced her own descent into the underworld. Near Isobel's Chiron return, her mother became sick, and she needed around-the-clock care before she died. Isobel was estranged from her mother but wanted to help her sister. She begrudgingly packed her bags and flew home.

It was a painful process for her; she'd never forgiven her mother for rejecting her when she came out. At first, she felt angry and resentful, seething with animosity each day as she cared for her. But after a few weeks, as she watched her mother's body wane, something began to shift. She started to see her mom as weak and humble as opposed to the villainous bully she had once been. Her mom's fighting spirit morphed into a gentle disposition full of humility and grace. The two of them began to bond. It was a sweet time for Isobel. She felt close to her mother in a way she hadn't since she was a child.

Within a few weeks, though, her mother died.

Isobel's grieving process became all-encompassing. She mourned her mother, but she also mourned the time lost, the years they spent angry and avoidant. She vacillated between sadness and rage, still upset at her mother for rejecting her. It was a lot for Isobel, who was also going through menopause then too.

It took Isobel many months to begin to find coherence around this experience. To do so, she needed to isolate from others and be alone. Like a molting snake shedding her skin, she felt vulnerable and raw. It was disorienting. Normally she felt confident, in charge, and capable. But now she was on the edge of a moral, existential crisis. She realized her exterior personality had covered up this deeper pain within, and she could no longer conjure that side of herself. However, her mother had left her a house and some money. With it, Isobel invested in some trainings. First reiki, which served as a gateway into the metaphysical world, something she always had felt judgmental toward. She eventually went back to school, to train in depth psychology, and now she supports people in their own healing journey by helping them reach beyond the facade of their identity and access a deeper truth within. While she's still sad about her lost years with her mother, she feels connected to a purpose she didn't have before.

Chiron in Your Natal Chart: Putting It to Work for You

Chiron's story is one of my favorites. This story reveals another dimension of our natal Chiron sign: where we are meant to journey through our anguish in order to help facilitate the healing of others. Although we may face difficulty in healing ourselves, we can often use it to cultivate wisdom and lend guidance to those who experience something similar. Chiron, who was as inherently (and beautifully) flawed as we are, stayed devoted to the healing of others; so can you, and so can all of us. This is another way we transform our trauma and sensitivities into our greatest gifts.

As he dances between Saturn's and Uranus's orbits, Chiron integrates the energies of its neighbor planets by teaching us to lean into lifelong revolutions of struggle — the experience of our wounds — and break free to rebirth healthier versions of ourselves.

Chiron's time in each sign varies. (He spends as little as two years in some signs and as much as eight years in others.) When Chiron is activated in your chart, you may have experiences that force you to confront why you are here on this inspiring yet sometimes challenging planet. In doing so, you cultivate compassion for yourself and the suffering of all beings.

FINDING YOUR CHIRON PLACEMENT

Given that astrology dates back thousands of years, Chiron's discovery four-plus decades ago is recent. Since Chiron isn't a planet, and he is fairly new, his placement isn't always indicated on computer-generated astrological charts. As instructed throughout the book, the free companion *Cosmic Health* ebook will direct you to a reputable place to obtain a chart, with instructions on how to make sure Chiron is included. To learn more, please go to Jennifer Racioppi.com/resources.

The following is a summary of each Chiron placement, indicating the nature of each placement's impact and opportunity for deeper empathy:

Chiron in Aries ♈

Your Chiron Message: With Chiron in Aries (cardinal fire), you might feel like it's hard to get your way. Or that when you try to step into a role of leadership your authority is undermined. Here's the deal: you are here to learn sovereignty and how to self-authorize without needing approval from others.

Your Empathetic Superpower: You have the capacity to understand other people's insecurities, especially when it comes to risk-taking. You also embody a deep compassion for others' anger and frustration.

Chiron in Taurus ♉

Your Chiron Message: With Chiron in Taurus (fixed earth), using your voice and speaking your truth may feel scary. Early in life you might experience a sense of there not being "enough." Yet your challenge is to push through your resistance to pleasure and nurture yourself, regardless. Most importantly, learn to love, trust, and nourish your body.

Your Empathetic Superpower: You have incredible insight into how to nourish others. You can anticipate their needs in advance, but really you are here to teach others about embodiment — how to be grounded and secure within themselves.

Chiron in Gemini ♊

Your Chiron Message: With Chiron in Gemini (mutable air), you might doubt your intellect or your ability to communicate your ideas, but you are actually quite adept at it. Journaling helps you to hear yourself think. Using affirmations to train your brain is helpful too.

Your Empathetic Superpower: You have an impeccable mind and an uncanny ability to hear wisdom and deliver it yourself. Most importantly, you understand that everyone has insecurities, and you create a safe container for people to share honestly.

Chiron in Cancer ♋

Your Chiron Message: With Chiron in Cancer (cardinal water), looking at the matrilineal line in your family will help you to better understand where forgiveness is required. You might not have been allowed to have feelings as a child. Learning how to feel safe and secure within yourself, at home in your body, is key.

Your Empathetic Superpower: You have a nourishing touch that soothes others. People come to you to feel connected and loved. You have an uncanny ability to help people feel seen, heard, recognized, and understood. Your compassionate heart can empathize with all, ranging from people without homes, to those who feel abandoned, to anyone suffering from body-image issues.

Chiron in Leo ♌

Your Chiron Message: With Chiron in Leo (fixed fire), you may feel reticent when it comes to expressing yourself genuinely. Your childhood may have been disrupted and creativity left un-indulged. Or you suffer from a belief that play is frivolous. Your healing edge remains to learn how to indulge your creativity and express yourself. Look to the patrilineal line in your family to see where forgiveness can be offered.

Your Empathetic Superpower: You understand the importance of seeing and championing others. You have the capacity to instill confidence in those around you, encouraging them to rise above the limitations of their own inner critic and trust in their ability to grow, shine, and lead.

Chiron in Virgo ♍

Your Chiron Message: With Chiron in Virgo (mutable earth), you may have suffered from health issues that held you back. You can be very self-critical, but developing a strong spiritual practice helps you to surrender to the divine and, in doing so, take (some) pressure off yourself.

Your Empathetic Superpower: You are a gifted healer. You help others access the sovereignty within to establish the boundaries they need to care for themselves, especially as it relates to learning to slow down and integrate mindfulness and self-compassion into their lives.

Chiron in Libra ♎

Your Chiron Message: With Chiron in Libra (cardinal air), it's easy to fall into codependent relationships or dynamics where you feel obliged to align with others for safety. Learning how to establish healthy boundaries, and even more importantly how to say no, liberates you. But the real work is in finding the ability to say yes to you.

Your Empathetic Superpower: You have an astute ability to be both fair and balanced. You fight for the underdog and know how to deeply empathize with others. You are driven toward justice, and you fight on behalf of liberation for all. You are here to champion new ways of being in the world that are anti-oppressive in nature.

Chiron in Scorpio ♏

Your Chiron Message: With Chiron in Scorpio (fixed water), chances are you suffered a betrayal early in life that causes you to mistrust others. Sexually, you may feel shy or challenged. Learning how to integrate your sexuality as a divine part of you and an integral facet of life brings healing—but this is challenging.

Your Empathetic Superpower: You understand the hesitation to share secrets and can help build intimacy with others by establishing trust. You have a strong capacity to keep confidences, and you excel in the role of the therapist, investigator, or friend.

Chiron in Sagittarius ♐

Your Chiron Message: With Chiron in Sagittarius (mutable fire), you avoid blunt honesty. Learning how to listen to and honor your own raw truth is a must. In doing so, you transcend dogma and live your potential, even finding freedom in your body, mind, and heart.

Your Empathetic Superpower: You embody the archetype of the teacher. You have a natural capacity to help others own their own wisdom, pursue freedom, and speak their truth. You are here on behalf of liberation.

Chiron In Capricorn ♑

Your Chiron Message: With Chiron in Capricorn (cardinal earth), you are here to undo the impact and legacy of oppressive patriarchal practices. While at times you may not feel sovereign yourself, pursuing your own authority is critical.

Your Empathetic Superpower: You know how to support others in accessing their inner guide. You are here to help others establish boundaries, undo overachieving, and honor their bodies. You teach them the power of reclaiming the right to be and disrupting oppressive power dynamics.

Chiron in Aquarius ♒

Your Chiron Message: With Chiron in Aquarius (fixed air), you are not here to fit in but instead to forge your own path. You are here to push back against the belief systems of culture, society, and your family to support the birth of a new paradigm. The challenge is that you can at times feel like an outcast or orphaned.

Your Empathetic Superpower: Because you are ahead of your time, and you know what it's like to feel like an outcast, you have an astute understanding of how to help others feel seen, heard, and witnessed.

Chiron in Pisces ♓

Your Chiron Message: With Chiron in Pisces (mutable water), you have an incredible propensity toward empathy, but at times you may feel like a martyr or victim, hijacked by the needs, wants, and desires of others. Learning boundaries is incredibly important for you. At an early age you may have been shamed for being too sensitive, or even gifted psychically.

Your Empathetic Superpower: Because empathy is second nature to you, you have a notable capacity to anticipate the needs of others. Self-expression through art is healing. But truly, your empathetic superpower lies in your intuitive gifts. You can see, know, and feel with uncanny accuracy.

Chiron in Retrograde

As the astrological influence that enables us to evolve in spite of our core wound—a wound that we can neither erase nor fully heal—Chiron's retrograde asks us to elevate how that wound affects, and even facilitates, our personal and spiritual growth. When Chiron travels retrograde, we have an opportunity to see how and where we can use his lessons to cultivate and deepen our compassion.

The specific areas where we can offer more empathy and caring depend on the zodiac sign that Chiron is transiting. Generally speaking, since Chiron is an outer centaur, his retrograde does not always have obvious impacts on us. Still, his annual invitations to deepen our compassion, even for those whom we prefer to deny or shun, can deliver profound growth that ultimately allows us to support greater healing in our lives and our world.

Chiron Ritual: Embrace Your Creative Healing

Dealing with your core wound is a lifelong journey that may include different kinds of therapy. However, the power of a creative process is often underestimated on the path to healing. As we travel the bridge from Saturn to the transpersonal planets, there's no better ritual than one that involves art. Here are two to consider:

Cathartic Collaging

Collaging is a powerful way to process deeper emotions. The typical instructions for vision boards apply—glue, a pile of magazines, and poster board are all you need. I once did four smaller vision boards and collaged for each element—air, fire, water, and earth—to put myself in touch with my feelings about each one. That activated the healing essence of each element. You can try that as well or focus your collage on whatever you're feeling at a given moment. The idea is to tap into imagery, color, and emotions that allow you to process your feelings as they relate to the material covered in this chapter.

Playlist Your Way Through Pain

With so many streaming services, we all have more music available than the kings and queens of antiquity. Begin by streaming music that helps you to connect to your emotions or that matches your mood. Create a playlist and add songs that help you tell your story. We all have wounds; however, none of us has the same story. By using songs, create a playlist that takes you through the arc of your pain. When done well, this task can take several days. In the process, you'll discover new music, hear lyrics with fresh ears, and create a beautiful playlist that tells the story of your life, wound, and pain. Name your playlist accordingly. Come back and listen to it whenever you like. Listening to it with headphones helps since they provide the privacy that's often necessary for healing.

CHAPTER 14

Uranus

Authenticity and Breakthrough

From Chiron's kind-hearted, selfless ways, we enter Uranus's domain of eccentricity, disruption, revolution, and breakthrough.

As one of the transpersonal planets, Uranus is slow moving, taking approximately seven years to transit each zodiac sign, and eighty-four years to transit all twelve signs. As a result, Uranus affects generations and tends to influence broader cultural trends and movements as well as our personal experience.

Uranus was discovered in 1781, shortly after the start of the industrial revolution, and its equator is situated at an almost perfect right angle to its orbit. In keeping with its quirky nature, Uranus spins on its side, unlike any of the other planets in our solar system. Because of this, Uranus experiences the most extreme weather. For a quarter of its orbit, while the sun shines directly over each of its poles, the rest of the planet descends into dark winter—for twenty-one years.[1]

All of this is to say: Uranus stands out with unapologetic intensity.

Like his planetary tilt, Uranus does things differently, often turning things on their heads—and not gently or slowly, at that. His need for bone-deep truth and radical authenticity is undeniable, even brash. He demands that we step up and boldly face that which we might prefer to deny.

Unwilling to settle for less than what he knows we are capable of, Uranus won't hesitate to deliver disruption that can act as a powerful catalyst for change. When he strikes in this way, our job is to find our way through the chaos and, in the process, discover—and insist on—attaining new and purer levels of illumination.

Like Aquarius, the zodiac sign he calls home, Uranus is quirky, demanding, and revolutionary for good reason. He doesn't believe in change for change's sake. His endgame is always liberation—from the chains of our limiting beliefs and patterns, from the societal shoulds and have-tos that inform our traditions, assumptions, and biases, as well as from mental, emotional, physical, and spiritual constraints.

Uranus can feel like a wrecking ball creating havoc in our lives, derailing any and all illusions of security. Unwilling to hold back for anything or anyone, this planet has the capacity to shake our identity, values, and sense of reality to their very core.

When this happens, we may feel abandoned, even betrayed, but herein lies Uranus's lessons and his genius also. Like his transpersonal planetary friends Neptune and Pluto, he gives us more than we can handle, pushing our capacity to enter an entirely new realm of possibility. He challenges us to work through the inevitable upheavals of life and break free not just from the status quo but also from our attachment to beliefs that may be holding us back. Ultimately, Uranus calls to our most expressed and embodied creativity and freedom.

Uranus in Taurus (2018–2026): Reclaiming the Divine Feminine

Given Uranus's generational footprint, he is especially adept at transforming our societal structures and cultural belief systems.

In May 2018, Uranus moved into Taurus for the first time in seventy-seven years. Uranus dismantles power to birth innovation—we saw this during his previous transit in Aries from 2011 to 2018, a sign known as the independent trailblazer. During those years, we saw a revolution around personal identity, facilitated by the rise of social media. As a result of new technology, the personal brand came into being. After decades of conventional full-time employment being the only acceptable norm, suddenly new employment options, especially self-employment, presented themselves. I, myself, rode this wave. Twenty years ago, I would never have been able to build a robust international following doing what I do without television fame. Yet during that Uranus transit, I was able to build my business via blogging on a WordPress site. *So* Uranus in Aries!

Unlike Aries, which is ruled by Mars, Taurus is ruled by Venus. Venus relates to feminine energy, values, money, and relationships. As Uranus moves through Taurus, the sacred feminine will be redefined and resurrected in a new and revolutionary form. The seven years Uranus will be in Taurus will largely be about breaking down the barriers and limitations around what's possible for oppressed populations, embodied healing, and new ways of relating to Earth—a movement we already see.

The message? Watch out, patriarchy—the feminine is rising!

News flash: she's *not* a middle-class white woman. She's not even necessarily "female" in the traditional sense. This rise is intersectional, including the spectrum of gender identity as well as multiracial and socioeconomic diversity.

Uranus is a rule breaker and a revolutionary, so our gender norms will be transformed. For some, this may not feel comfortable—Uranus transits rarely do—even more so since Taurus is a stable, steady, Venus-ruled, fixed-earth sign. Uranus's disruption will unground the grounded. That means traditions will be challenged, dismantled, and reimagined. Amidst the routine and predictability Taurus is known for, Uranus will disrupt power dynamics that have limited us for millennia. While transiting Taurus, Uranus is likely to level the playing field for women, men, and nonbinary people, as well as anyone from historically marginalized identities, to reveal previously unmet potentials.

This process started to gain more consistent momentum in March 2019, when Uranus finished his dance between signs, which he often does when he enters a new zodiac sign. This particular "dance" looks like this:

May 2018 to November 2018: Uranus in Taurus
November 2018 to March 2019: Uranus in Aries
March 2019 to July 2025: Uranus in Taurus
July 2025 to November 2025: Uranus in Gemini
November 2025 to April 2026: Uranus will complete its journey in
    Taurus

Uranus in Taurus (2018–2026): Restoring Mother Earth

At the time of this book's release, Uranus will traverse the early degrees of Taurus. In addition to disrupting heteropatriarchal white supremacist norms we will simultaneously be called to restore Mother Earth.

As the planet that supports our very existence, Earth demands our attention as she continues to suffer rampant pollution and the loss of vital ecosystems, resulting in climate change. During this transit, we are having to face the radical truth about how we relate to our planet, our bodies, food, farming systems, money, and other material resources. We will be called to step up and do all that we can to rally behind her.

Uranus will help us, albeit not always in ways that feel gentle or easy. Whatever it takes, he will push protocols that further the restoration of our planet. This will include renegotiating how we individually and collectively relate to our resources and tend to Earth.

My personal passion for restoring our planet runs deep, and this is, without a doubt, among the more important and far-reaching potential effects of Uranus's transit through Taurus. By doing so, we can potentially break a spell that's shrouded this planet for hundreds of years.

As we have seen with the COVID-19 outbreak that first took the world by storm in early 2020, we live in a time riddled with disruption and chaos. This pandemic, which began when Jupiter, Saturn, and Pluto conjoined in Capricorn, demonstrated how quickly our everyday norms can be disrupted, and just how fragile human life and the resources and structures we rely on to survive really are. Yet even amidst tremendous global chaos, there are opportunities—for the planet to begin to heal and for us to adapt, ideally by creating a more sustainable and universally supportive society and way of life. This is the essence of Uranus's healing magic. His disruption isn't often easy, but through it, he offers us the opportunity to reemerge as more aware and evolved stewards of this planet and each other.

Making It Personal: Creating from Chaos

Uranus was the Greek god of the sky and heavens. He visited Gaia (Earth) every night to mate with her, and it was because of their nightly unions that the twelve Titans were born. However, Uranus was disgusted and threatened by his strong, enormous, multi-headed, multi-armed children, so he threw them into Tartarus, the deepest, darkest pit under the earth.

A loving mother, Gaia couldn't forgive her husband for his treatment of their children. After fashioning a sickle, she armed her Titan sons to get revenge on their father and liberate their brothers. All of Uranus's sons failed to carry out her mission except Cronus (Saturn), who stepped up and castrated Uranus. As Uranus's genitals fell into the sea, Aphrodite, the goddess of love, was born.

Once again, as with the creation story beginning with Chaos, the great void, love and beauty are created from chaos and destruction; birth mandates some form of death.

It's of course one thing to talk about the necessary role of destruction in every act of creation when it's mythology, mass culture, or theory. It's entirely another when this kind of mayhem is unleashed in our lives. How can we create something new when we're devastated emotionally, physically, spiritually, or otherwise? How can we create meaning when chaos is desecrating our very foundation?

When Uranus touches down in your chart via a transit, or if Uranus plays a dominant role in your natal chart, you may find yourself bucking norms in order to live in fuller alignment with your absolute truth. This is all-or-nothing territory, a zone where half-truths carry no weight. This instinct to take down the old and reinvent ourselves can serve us, helping us to detach from what has been and focus on creating something new.

I personally owe a huge thank-you to my Uranus placement (as well as my Saturn placement in my natal chart). While both planets shaped my cosmic curriculum in undeniable ways, Uranus's role holds extra weight.

For me, studying astrology was a way to heal and understand my radical hysterectomy, or female castration. Unlike with Uranus, my castration wasn't a punishment, yet still, the outcome was eerily reminiscent of his. Indeed, not comfortable or easy. However, I can now see that my illness served as an initiation of my soul and propelled me, unimaginably, in directions I could not otherwise reach. As harsh as that Uranian-type upheaval was in my body, spirit, and life, inner liberation is a powerful gift.

In a world where compromise is our default, when Uranus touches down in our lives, his uncompromising standards say "I tell no" to anything that's less than what is aligned with the essence of our soul. The truth is, Uranus demands we create from chaos and see Chaos as the goddess she is, the void preceding conception. And the universe we give birth to on the other side is fresh, new, alive, full of potential. (Our liberation demands no less.)

Claiming Your Right to Break Free

When Uranus becomes prominent in your chart, these are your moments to awaken hidden dreams and do things differently—with more truth, risk-taking, even rebellion and adventure. This is your call to drop the roles you are playing and reengage in the world with devotion to your truth. This is when you can reclaim your thirst for liberation and realize dreams that never before seemed possible.

Consider how Uranus transits map to your life:

Age twenty-one: Uranus squares your natal Uranus placement. For many, this is the end of formal education and entering socially recognized adulthood. Saturn brings on the responsibility; Uranus lends a spirit of freedom and exploration. We push the edge of what is possible.

Age forty-two: Uranus is opposite your natal Uranus placement. Typically, these are the years you might experience what is known as the classic midlife crisis. But really this transit transcends that trope! It has the potential to bring the ultimate liberation. It's a special time in life, offering a soul initiation to clear pain and bondage from the past—in both the psyche and the soma. It's about channeling the energy of quick-fire authenticity to defy the limits of assimilation, and finally, find yourself.

Age sixty-three: Uranus again squares your natal Uranus placement. Now well beyond the menopausal transition and fully in the power of the crone archetype, you have the capacity to channel your authenticity and light. There's little that can hold you back from claiming your sovereignty. This is a sacred period of life when you are charged with the task of reviewing your cosmic curriculum and reconciling where you still feel stifled.

Age eighty-four: Uranus returns to your natal Uranus placement. Uranus comes back to its zodiac sign at the time of your birth. This is a time to unapologetically embody who you are.

Given Uranus's broader generational and cultural impact, we also need to consider this from a sociopolitical perspective. Throughout history, horrific events have, at times, activated a previously dormant drive for knowledge, resource building, and unity. During tremendous hardship, we are often also pushed to do things differently, whether to protect ourselves or prevent devastation from recurring.

Just as a wide-scale crisis has the potential to bring about global solidarity, personal crisis can spur our internal solidarity. In our turmoil, we always have the opportunity to commit to our truth and hold our own hands in navigating the unknowns of a new, unfamiliar reality. We can rebel against what we've known, honor our right to liberation, and pursue our most embodied life with unapologetic intensity.

Facilitating Your Own (R)Evolution

In addition to bringing massive change, Uranus can encourage you to engage in seemingly small acts that don't initially seem rebellious or radical but end up being exactly that. Here are some ways to engage in your own Uranian (r)evolution.

Dare to Tell Your (Whole) Truth

Years ago, I attended a lecture on resilience taught by Dr. Maria Sirois and Mark Matousek in a church in New York City. I knew Maria's teachings well but had never heard Mark speak. During that talk, he had everyone in the room open up a notebook and write down all the little lies we were telling ourselves—that our emotions don't matter, that we're happy when we're really not, and so on. He said that tackling that list was the first step to coming into a deeper sense of resilience.

His message was clear and concise: resilience requires authenticity. Mark's teaching that night felt like a lesson in Uranus 101: tell yourself the truth, at all costs.

As the twelve-step recovery adage goes, "We're only as sick as our secrets." Uranus insists that we become radically honest. This naked honesty is at the heart of the revolution he urges us to wage.

Find the Opportunity

In chapter 1 we discussed rose-colored realism. This begins with telling the truth, which we've now done, but that's not an end goal unto itself. Uranus ultimately aims to liberate us in new ways.

That liberation may be a radical reinvention of your identity after a divorce, or after becoming a mom. Or maybe you're seeking love, yearning to have a child, or starting a different career. Maybe your opportunity appears through a break from a previous attachment: your children leaving for college, a parent passing away, or the loss of a job.

Each of these is an opportunity for liberation through the disruption of the status quo. While you can and should mourn loss in your life, you must eventually also consider how to spend your mornings now that you don't need to get your kids to school. Released from the corporate hustle, will you strike out on your own or explore a radically new career field? No longer tethered to an unhappy marriage, how will you look, feel, laugh, love, and live?

Build Your Support System

Since Uranus is also the ruler of Aquarius—who naturally corresponds with the eleventh house, which is traditionally associated with friendship—Uranus brings an inherent emphasis on groups, organizations, acquaintances, and also our ability to realize desires.

Connect with loved ones and consider other ways you might build, or activate, your support system. Also consider how else you might equip yourself. What knowledge do you need to navigate your new reality? What skills might you look to build?

Be Committed to Your Self-Discovery

Complement your action with introspection. Notice how your reinvention manifests externally as well as internally. Stay curious and open to new ways of moving forward, of integrating what is unfolding around you and within you.

Integrating Reinvention

Although Uranus, which is always at a tilt, does ask us to flip the script, he does not want us to find a new way to mask who we are just because it's different. Remember, this is revolution and upheaval with a purpose — to awaken to a new level of our authenticity, and in so doing, to become more liberated, so you are ready and able to serve the greater good.

In these times of rebuilding, we must lean on our true essence more than ever, but not disregard the past or reject who we are. In the process of Uranus-inspired reinvention, it is important to remember that we are not called to change who we are at our core but to reevaluate whether we are living in alignment with that core.

Authenticity — the act of living in reflection of our true personality, beliefs, and values — is a fundamentally necessary practice. Consider the harm we do to ourselves when we suppress our true selves. We are basically telling ourselves that we do not have the agency, right, or acceptance to show who we really are. This can affect our health as well; inauthenticity has been shown to cause feelings of immorality and impurity.[2] Conversely, authenticity contributes to increased self-esteem, subjective well-being, and psychological well-being.[3] While we have a desire to belong, it is a distinctly human need to stand out and live in accordance with our truth.

Standing out can also feel scary, even isolating. Being authentic and living authentically, especially when doing so requires massive change, may at times turn people off. While radical authenticity is not always possible, practical, or beneficial, people-pleasing can also become a habit that seems safer, as it often provides some level of social inclusion, acceptance, and gratification. However, that external validation ultimately comes at a cost to your truth and your health. While the edgier sides of you may not appeal to or agree with everyone else, they powerfully define aspects of who you are. By not suppressing those parts of yourself, you'll eventually find the people who do appreciate, accept, and support you at your most authentic.

Using Our Collective Voice

As we evolve into more authentic versions of ourselves and connect with our people, Uranus also asks us to consider our collective voice. How are we expressing ourselves on the world stage? Consider your Saturn-inspired purpose—is there a bigger social or cultural movement that resonates with you?

When we act in concert with like-minded people, we channel our individual voices into a collective whole that can make big things happen. Consider the massive transformations—sometimes for better, sometimes for worse—that we experience because of social movements. The election of world leaders, dictatorial takeovers, climate justice, civil rights, policy reform, cultural revolutions. These all fall under Uranus's (sometimes volatile, yet ultimately constructive) correlative domain.

CAN SOCIAL ACTIVISM IMPROVE HEALTH HABITS?

In 2012, Megan E. Gilster performed research on the benefits of volunteering and activism, finding that the psychological benefits of well-being and social connection associated with volunteering were also present with activism. However, activism added the additional benefit of empowerment.[4]

In her 2018 research for her PhD dissertation, Elizabeth Emley found that involvement in a social movement acts as a "stealth intervention" for increasing health-oriented behaviors, including more nutritious eating and physical movement.[5]

This intersection of health outcomes and activism is an emerging focus for researchers, but so far what evidence points to is this: contributing to a greater cause, spurred by connection and collaboration with others, provides a deeply intrinsic motivation to align our behaviors with our core values, with those who support that cause. Also, since social-change movements are often directed toward eliminating systemic oppression, which contributes to poor health, those cause-promoting behaviors bolster additional health outcomes.

Plus, with the emerging call for activists to practice self-care in the name of social change—emphasizing recovery and introspection—we have entered a reality in which activism is not synonymous with sacrifice and eternal burnout.

Uranus: It's All About Freedom

Before I close out this chapter on Uranus, I'd be remiss if I didn't throw you a curveball. It's Uranus, after all. There's another point of view to consider when digesting who Uranus is and the role he plays in astrology. According to one of the leading authorities in both astrology and cultural history, Uranus was misnamed. Scholar Richard Tarnas offers another interpretation of who Uranus is. He believes Uranus's archetype aligns more fully to Prometheus than with the mythology of his namesake.

He writes in his book *Prometheus the Awakener: An Essay on the Archetypal Meaning of the Planet Uranus:*

I had been conscious of this discrepancy for some time when I noticed that those same astrological qualities fit another figure in Greek Mythology with extraordinary precision. This figure was Prometheus, the titan who rebelled against the gods, helped overthrow tyrannical Kronos, tricked Zeus, and stole fire from Mount Olympus to liberate humanity from god's power. Prometheus was considered the wisest of his race and taught humankind all the arts and sciences. The more I examined the matter, the more I realized that every quality astrologers associate with Uranus was reflected in the myth of Prometheus: the initiation of radical change, the passion for freedom, the defiance of authority, the act of cosmic rebellion against a universal structure to free humanity of bondage, the urge to transcend limitation, the intellectual brilliance and genius, the element of excitement and risk.[6]

Remember Chiron's story? Born as a centaur and abandoned as a child, he grew up to make significant contributions as a healer and teacher, becoming famous for his gifts, his contributions to medicine, and his ability to raise heroes. Struck with a deadly arrow that caused a wound he could neither heal nor be relieved of through death because of his immortality, Chiron lived with immense physical and psychological pain while devoting himself to healing others. It was Prometheus who he traded his immortality to save. Chiron liberated Prometheus, in turn liberating himself from his own immortality. But Prometheus also liberated Chiron and then went on to liberate the world.

Take that in. Chiron—half man, half horse, destined to live a life of pain for eternity, but committed to excellence through his knowledge, talent, skill, and empathy—gave up his life so Prometheus could level the playing field between the gods and humanity.

It's important to see Uranus's impact in our lives, and in the world, as the path to liberation.

Uranus in Your Natal Chart: Putting It to Work for You

Uranus's placement in your chart indicates where you're called to stir the pot and pursue personal (r)evolution.

Uranus in Aries ♈: You are here to disrupt the status quo by being you. Authenticity is your key word. Innovate through individuation.

Uranus in Taurus ♉: You are here to disrupt practices that are not aligned with supporting the environment, the collective liberation of humanity, or healing the earth.

Uranus in Gemini ♊: You are here to innovate as a communicator and networker. Having a broad and diverse social community remains essential.

Uranus in Cancer ♋: You are here to disrupt patriarchal traditions as well as motherhood and family patterns.

Uranus in Leo ♌: You are here to disrupt the status quo by bringing ingenuity to play, creativity, and business, leading in dynamic and effective ways.

Uranus in Virgo ♍: You are here to innovate with regard to work–life balance, health, diet, and ways you relate to the environment.

Uranus in Libra ♎: You are here to innovate relationship dynamics. You have a unique way of weaving beauty into your home and your sense of style, and perhaps you are an artist. Above all, you are here on behalf of equality.

Uranus in Scorpio ♏: You bring new dimensions of spirituality, financial management, and sex to life. You are unafraid of exploring the shadows in your soul.

Uranus in Sagittarius ♐: You are here to disrupt power dynamics that limit freedom. You bring new ways of relating to religion, philosophy, and thinking.

Uranus in Capricorn ♑: You are here to disrupt the status quo of business as usual, bringing innovation to work in pursuit of dismantling hierarchies.

Uranus in Aquarius ♒: You are here as a rebel and a leader, building a new paradigm based on humanitarian values.

Uranus in Pisces ♓: You innovate in the realms of spirituality and art. You are here to disrupt dogma and martyrdom, and to liberate your intuitive knowing.

Uranus in Retrograde

As the planet most closely associated with authenticity, awakening, and liberation, Uranus retrograde asks us to integrate the sometimes sudden, unexpected lessons we've learned in these areas. As a slower-moving outer planet, Uranus reverses each year by about four degrees over a period of approximately five months. This gives us an opportunity to look at how we've evolved in the cosmic area(s) Uranus is transiting and take the necessary action to assimilate those lessons.

During Uranus retrograde, we're called to look inward—inside ourselves and inside the fabric and structure of our society, economy, and more. The particular focus of this introspective yet proactive period depends on the zodiac sign and degrees that Uranus is retrograding through that year.

Above all, Uranus retrograde asks us to look at where we feel an urge to break free, be more authentic, and take action that liberates us from norms that feel stifling and/or stagnant. By making relevant changes in these areas, we ready ourselves to evolve further once Uranus stations direct.

Journal Your Radical Truth

We all hide from truths in our lives. I'm not referring to obvious lies but rather to the hidden truths we may never admit to anyone—including ourselves. In a journal, answer the question "What lie am I telling myself?" Without forcing yourself to resolve it, freewrite your truth at length, allowing yourself to release any stuck emotions it brings up. Keep writing, filling three or more handwritten pages, recording your thoughts and feelings as you do. Taking this small but important action is cathartic unto itself.

Uranus Ritual: It's all about the Fire, Baby. Steal It Back!

This ritual serves as a bridge, taking you from where you've been and moving you into your intended future. It helps you integrate the lessons you have learned from Saturn, Chiron, Uranus, and Prometheus. In this ritual you will connect with the archetypes associated with the celestial bodies we are working with. While you can do this ritual anytime you are ready, no matter the moon phase, it's most ideally done when the moon is in a fire sign, waxing between the new moon and full moon.

Before beginning this ritual, you may want to repeat the cosmic bath in the Full Moon Ritual (see chapter 5). This will center you and prepare you, but it's not a required step; this ritual is powerful regardless.

To begin this ritual, you need some simple items:

- Your journal
- Two white candles
- One red candle
- An old key that you no longer need
- A small sachet

When you are ready, take a seated position at your altar. Gently lower your eyelids and connect with your inner cosmos, the universe within. Take a moment to light the white candles. Once they are lit, you are ready to begin.

Consider the following myths and archetypes. One at a time, connect with each.

Prometheus: the liberator and the warrior
Chiron: the wounded and the healer
Saturn: the teacher and the disciplinarian
Uranus: the revolutionary and the disruptor

In your journal, answer the following questions:

- *How do I relate to these archetypes, if at all?*
- *Which one do I feel most drawn to?*

Think about each archetype individually and ask yourself, "What can I learn from them?"

Now turn your attention to Chiron specifically and ask yourself these questions:

- *What experiences have brought me great pain?*
- *What have those same experiences taught me?*
- *How can I integrate these healing lessons?*

As you write out your answers, be specific and detail oriented. If you created a playlist, as mentioned in the previous chapter, this is a wonderful time to listen to it.

Take a moment. Put your hand on your heart, and center yourself. Send yourself loving-kindness, as though you were witnessing your best friend. Out loud, give yourself a nurturing reflection. Name your strengths. Go back to the mantra you created at the end of chapter 7 and recite it to yourself.

Write a list of all the ways you feel you've grown because of these experiences. How have they helped you to become more empathetic, wise, and capable of helping others?

Now let's focus on Chiron's glyph for a moment: ⚷. It looks like a key. Many astrologers believe — myself included — that Chiron holds the key to unlocking your healing magic.

Take the key on your altar and see it as a symbolic representation of what Chiron unlocks for you. How does your experience of Chiron help you to unlock your healing magic?

If you have a clear answer, take the key and place it somewhere sacred. You may even want to get a necklace for it and wear it as a reminder.

If you don't have a clear answer, take the key and put it in your sachet. Before going to bed at night, put it under your pillow with the intention of connecting to your understanding of your personal connection to Chiron in your sleep. Upon waking, journal immediately and see what wisdom comes through for you. Repeat this until you start to gain a sense of awareness about how Chiron helps you to unlock your healing magic.

Now it's time to steal back your fire. Connect with Prometheus and his story. He stole fire from the gods to liberate humanity and was then severely punished, until Chiron gave up his immortality so he could be released.

Who are the metaphorical "gods" keeping your fire? How will you steal your fire back? Spend as much time as you need journaling your answers.

Really think about this. Who has stolen your fire? What has stolen your fire? Continue to journal.

Now make a commitment to stealing it back. Get crystal clear on the action you can take to reignite your own flame, so you can take your fire back.

When you are ready, light the remaining, red candle. As you do, visualize your liberation. What tyranny are you freeing yourself from, by reclaiming your passion? Once you feel complete, you can begin to bring your ritual to completion.

As you close, acknowledge yourself and the archetypes we explored. Then say, "Thank you." Gently extinguish the white candles, however; assuming you are not immediately leaving your home and it's safe, allow the flame of your red candle to continue to burn.

CHAPTER 15

Neptune

Intuition and Spiritual Development

From Uranus's sudden and shocking jolts, we venture into watery Neptune and his ethereal, chimerical otherworld. Neptune, also known as Poseidon, god of the sea, is the ruler of Pisces. His focus is engaging mystical attunement, intuition, devotion, and nuance. Like Uranus, Neptune is a transcendental planet that has broader cultural and generational impacts, yet he can also affect our lives and our health in deep and powerful ways.

The Mysterious Realm

In 2017, while pursuing my dream to write a book, I had a very Neptunian moment that has had powerful ripple effects ever since. It was a weekday in summer, and I was on my way to a meeting with a major publisher to discuss the potential of this book. While driving into Manhattan for the meeting, I did what I often do and put on music. On that particular day, I'd chosen an album called *Planetarium*, which has a separate song for each planet. It begins with Neptune, which makes sense astrologically since Neptune rules music. The music is beautiful, alternately inspiring and haunting with an occasional trancelike quality. Listening to it, I felt a surge of inspiration. I got a flash of how I wanted to structure this book—I wanted to go through the planets one at a time, chapter by chapter, just as the *Planetarium* album does with its songs.

The meeting went well, so I began developing my idea, though I was advised not to pitch the book I'd envisioned and instead to focus on a concept considered to be more commercially viable. In perfect cosmic order, that attempt ultimately failed. A little over a year later, I signed a contract with a different publisher, who very much supported the book I yearned to write—precisely the book you now hold in your hands or hear through your headphones.

That brief burst of inspiration, that fleeting sense of intuitive knowing, is quintessential Neptune in a few important ways. In keeping with Neptune's spiritual, almost dreamlike nature, the message I received was primarily an intuitive one. I didn't have facts or figures to back up my inner knowing; I just sensed that my book idea was the right one. Also, my realization didn't arrive verbally. It came through music, which, for Neptune, is a source of healing and inspiration. Lastly, my intuitive knowing focused on topics that unto themselves are also very Neptune: astrology, spirituality, mysticism, and the psyche.

Neptune presents us with our inner underworld—the depths of our souls and the intangible knowing we gain from sources we can only sometimes pinpoint. Neptune's force beckons us inward, toward our most spiritual selves and a path of understanding oneness, harmony, beauty, and a connection to that which exists beyond the five senses.

Under Neptune's influence, we can access healing when we step away from a constant focus on the practical and tangible. He delivers inspiration and influences dreams, psychic receptivity, illusion, intuition, and spirituality.

Healing from Our Depths

From a cosmic health perspective, Neptune calls attention to our immune system and reminds us that nurturing the spiritual self is as critical to our health as tending to the physical body. In many ways we intuitively accept this idea that spirituality and the subconscious affect our health—that, for instance, we're more prone to getting sick when we're stressed beyond a healthy threshold. At the same time, however, we tend to downplay the importance of spirituality when we're healing the body or tending to other, seemingly unrelated parts of our lives.

Yet the central role of spirituality in our healing shows up repeatedly in ongoing research. Studies show that a consistent yoga practice can reduce pro-inflammatory markers in the body. (Specifically, one study showed that interleukin-1 beta cytokine levels were reduced.[1]) Meditation has also been shown to strengthen the immune system, increasing disease-fighting antibodies and reducing inflammation in older adults, corporate employees, even HIV patients.[2]

We see this same positive ripple effect in those who adhere to traditional faith practices, including regular attendance of religious services and prayer. People who report higher spirituality possess greater hope, anticipate pleasant events, experience less depression and anxiety, and have a lower risk of mortality. They're also more likely to turn to meditation than addictive substances or unhealthy behaviors in times of stress.[3] Remembrance of God (however you define it), or other spiritual forces we may believe in, buffers the impact of stress, allowing us to surrender to what is occurring and rely on a greater force to guide us toward resolution. Because of this, spirituality helps us to cope during challenging times, which then builds our resilience.

Spirituality also gives us a belief system and cohesive framework that provides meaning and a rationale for life's greatest phenomena and mysteries as well as the daily events that affect so much of our lives. In this sense, spirituality plays a key role in our human need for coherence and even order—a framework for living well morally and pro-socially.

These same principles apply to astrology, a spiritual practice that helps us relate to ourselves through the logic of the planets. Remember at the very beginning of this book when I discussed the interconnectivity of the universe and how we're each here to learn our cosmic curriculum? Astrology gives us a framework for navigating our experiences and understanding that even our greatest challenges can add depth and meaning to our lives. That relieves stress and anxiety that could otherwise wreak havoc on our immune system, and therefore our health.

There is a caveat to all of this, however. We're more likely to experience the positive health outcomes of our spiritual practice when we take an internal approach to it. Studies find that those who believe in and practice their religion as an aim in itself (internal orientation) experience better mental health and less depression and anxiety than those who use religion as a means for support, security, self-justification, social position, and more (external orientation).[4]

This emphasis on spirituality as a healing tool falls squarely within Neptune's realm. He comes to remind us of the immense importance of our spiritual beliefs and practices. Whatever our leanings, Neptune asks us to drop any dogmatic baggage we may be carrying, embody our sage-like wisdom, and embrace a softer and more open relationship with spirituality.

The Role of Sleep and Dreaming

As the ruler of the subconscious and our dreams, Neptune also highlights the importance of our most accessible gateway to these invisible yet paramount parts of ourselves: sleep.

With about a third of our lives devoted to slumbering, sleep is essential to our mental and physiological recovery and development. A good night's rest is linked to improved memory and critical thinking; longer life span; lower risk of cardiovascular disease, diabetes, and stroke; reduced stress and depression; and more balanced metabolism and weight. While I personally prefer eight to nine hours of sleep each night, some evidence suggests that six to seven hours is the sweet spot.[5]

When I first met her, Katya, an Asian woman, was a thirty-six-year-old professional in desperate need of the healing that comes from improved sleep. Suffering from painful periods and challenging premenstrual dysphoric disorder (PMDD), she felt overwhelmed by anxiety as well as painful bloating and digestive issues. From one day to the next, her moods were all over the place, going from extreme emotional highs to equally intense lows that included frequent crying spells. This was reflected in her chart as well. With a Pisces sun and Scorpio moon and rising signs, she had a lot of emotional depth and a fundamental need for intimacy that wasn't being met, leaving her vulnerable to her darker emotions, even victimhood. Feeling increasingly depressed, she began to doubt her inherent value. All of this was contributing to her chronic insomnia, which then exacerbated her other symptoms.

I suggested we begin with some health remedies, one of which was prioritizing sleep hygiene. This meant getting outside for at least thirty minutes every day to support her body's circadian rhythm, plus supplementing with a high dose of vitamin D (2,000 IU) in the morning to suppress melatonin production and optimize daytime hours. She also added low-impact movement to her morning routine. Each evening, she gave herself a laptop and digital device curfew, since blue light interferes with sleep, and took a hot shower before bed. Finally, she began tracking her sleep cycles, her emotions, and the phases of the moon to pinpoint periods of the lunar cycle where she needed to pay closer attention to her emotional needs.

Within weeks, Katya's sleep, energy, emotions, and digestion began to stabilize. Most important, by focusing on sleep hygiene, she allowed her body to heal and resume its natural cycle, which helped to regulate her emotions as well.

SOME OF MY FAVORITE SLEEP TIPS

These are my favorite ways to improve the length and quality of sleep:

- Get outside into sunlight during the day.
- Fit movement into your day — a sedentary lifestyle contributes to restless nights.
- Reduce or eliminate alcohol consumption.
- Restrict caffeine in the afternoon and evening.
- An hour or so before bedtime, drink soothing herbal tea, including blends specifically designed for bedtime.
- Take calming supplements before bed. Here are some that are known to support sleep: magnesium glycinate, CBD, 5-HTP (5-hydroxytryptophan), melatonin, valerian, magnolia, kava, skullcap, GABA (gamma-aminobutyric acid), and holy basil.
- Take a hot shower. Gently massage your body afterward using a soothing oil or lotion.
- Give yourself a foot massage with castor oil and a few drops of lavender oil.
- Have an orgasm before bed, which helps you relax.
- Install blackout window shades in your bedroom.
- Use a nighttime eye mask to block ambient light.
- Eat lightly at night, especially before bed.
- Gently stretch or meditate.
- Journal before bedtime, reflecting and savoring your moments of gratitude.

The Healing Rewards of the Dream State

Beyond its hallmark contributions to physical and mental health, sleep activates creative thinking and problem-solving. In a 2017 *TIME Special Edition* article, Harvard University psychologist Deirdre Barrett explained that when we sleep, "the brain thinks much more visually and intuitively."[6] While in your conscious state, the brain blocks thoughts that are deemed inappropriate, both socially and contextually. During sleep, your occipital lobes (visual centers) amp up. Information travels more freely between left and right brain hemispheres, all working to unleash the imagination. Again, we're reminded that the seeming nonsense of our deeper realms—which in this case means our dreams—may in fact be the doorway to our genius.

Since dreams often communicate key concepts and ideas, I recommend getting your z's with a pad and pen near your bed. You'll experience your more memorable dreams during the REM phase of sleep; this typically occurs during the last four hours of sleep, so prioritize getting those full nights rather than interrupted dozing.[7] If you wake up with a vivid awareness of your dreams, try to write down anything you remember. You may be fascinated by what your brain is processing at night. Dreams are another form of catharsis, a way for your brain to digest information and experiences that can't easily be processed during wakefulness.

In a world that's increasingly prioritizing productivity over recovery, we too often cheat sleep. Instead of turning off the light earlier, we stay up late or bring our devices to bed to respond to emails and peruse social media. Ironically, this "get more done" mentality degrades the length and quality of our sleep, which is at least as essential to our daytime productivity as our waking hours. Neptune says, "Enough"—and in fact, our health and well-being depend on it. In addition to increasing mortality risk, insufficient sleep over long periods of time has been shown to increase the risk of Alzheimer's disease later in life.[8] A recent study at Boston University found that the opposite is also true—sufficient deep sleep helps the brain to ward off dementia. The brain waves that occur during deep sleep act as cleaning agents, removing toxins from the brain that are known to contribute to Alzheimer's and other neurodegenerative diseases.[9]

OPTIMIZE YOUR SLEEP BY THE LUNAR PHASES

One of the coolest things I've learned through my years of working with astrology is that my sleep cycles are affected by the moon's phases. The full moon tends to interrupt my sleep, or it can make falling asleep harder. I've learned to accept this. I also sometimes use full moons to work late, indulge my creativity, and socialize more at night. Additionally, at the time of the full moon, I tend to crave different foods or have different digestive responses. Conversely, at the new moon, I get more restful sleep, my body's cravings feel more congruent, and I derive pleasure from more monastic practices. Try tracking how you sleep during the different phases of the moon and see what you discover.

The Medicinal Power of Music and Creativity

Under Neptune's guidance, nonverbal healing—through listening to music as well as creative expression—acts as a powerful salve. Pythagoras, an ancient Greek philosopher, developed an idea called *musica universalis* (universal music), or the "music of the spheres," which connected mathematics and sound. Everything, after all, is vibration and we can attune to these vibrations as a healing force. There are so many ways to heal, and many of them are more readily available than we realize.

There's a great deal of healing potential in immersing ourselves in music, especially when it lures us into a meditative state. The cathartic effects of music play out in the body as well as the mind. Listening to music offers similar health benefits to getting adequate sleep: sharpening learning and memory, boosting energy and happiness, moderating appetite through its calming effects, and promoting the release of dopamine, which counteracts stress.[10]

I credit my love of music and my community within the music world for helping me up-level my enjoyment of life. By appreciating music, I open my mind and connect to the music within. It's a spiritual practice that encourages me to consider the endless possibilities of life.

Some science even suggests there's more to it than that. In *The Body Keeps the Score*, author Bessel van der Kolk talks about "the healing power of community as expressed in music and rhythms."[11] When we synchronize with melody, we can also elevate our mood, change our breathing, and motivate ourselves to move the body more. With all of this in mind, I make sure to honor my "rocking out" time as much as I do my commitment to healthy eating and regular exercise.

Although I focus on music here, you also can use other arts to bring your dreams into reality while simultaneously processing your more earthly emotions. Artistic pursuits are a powerful way to give yourself a much-needed time-out from physical reality—you can dance, paint, write, or draw your way back to emotional equilibrium.

Neptune's Shadow: Vulnerability or Victimhood

While Neptune's trance can be enchanting, pulling us into the rhythms of nonverbal healing and imaginative and intuitive wandering, it can also create confusion.

Neptune's illusory side is especially important since it can be one of the most difficult when it comes to health. Its influence tends to be extreme, and its shadow can reveal where we're trying to escape from reality rather than heal. Under Neptune's shadow, creative illusions become destructive delusions. This is also the planet associated with deception, addiction, denial, and naiveté.

I view addiction, in all of its forms, to be a misappropriation of devotion. We stay devoted to the patterns, behaviors, foods, and people that hold us back from reaching our higher selves. If we flip that script and devote ourselves to our health, a higher purpose, music, art, love, and magic, we gain a very different perspective on just about everything in our lives.

So many facets of our health get derailed when we become complicit with addictions. Some addictions are easier to recognize, like dependence on drugs or alcohol. Others are less obvious, including our culturally normalized addictions to sugar, salt, and fatty foods as well as social media, shopping, work, caffeine, overscheduling ourselves, codependency, and more.

Left unchecked, Neptune can also call forth the victim archetype from within, convincing us to forsake the power we each hold to influence our health, well-being, and other parts of our lives. We've all experienced the victim archetype at some point, whether through codependency or the idea that no matter what we do we are doomed. This is Neptune at its worst, putting us in a trancelike state in which we surrender our innate power. When this illusion strikes, step back and notice it, and above all, maintain your agency. It is so important to recognize and respect your ability to create the change you desire.

Penny, a multiracial woman, began to appreciate the importance of reclaiming her agency during our time working together. When I first met her, she was recently divorced and mourning her marriage, but she also recognized the aspects of herself she'd denied in order to be the devoted partner and professional she'd thought her ex wanted her to be. While her melancholy marriage had provided for her financially, she'd never felt free, happy, or fulfilled. As the child of an alcoholic, she also hadn't yet made peace with the pain caused by her father's addiction. With her marriage now ending, she was finally able to grieve the childhood she'd never had, the marriage she'd lost, and the children she had wanted to have.

As a Sagittarius sun sign, Cancer moon, and Libra rising, she had a need for a healthy, interdependent partnership. Getting involved in Al-Anon helped her work through important aspects of her childhood and marriage. Going to therapy also proved essential, giving her the personalized support she most needed. Through this process she got back in touch with herself and her own power, and also reclaimed her love of art. Drawing, painting, and collage work were things she had let go of in college, when she first had set her sights on a corporate career. By bringing expressive arts back into her life, she was able to process emotions and reclaim the parts of her spirit she'd forgotten she needed.

Here are some general but important ways to work with Neptune:

- **Listen to music as a form of meditation.** Peruse your favorite music-streaming service for new options or listen to vinyl — it sounds better. You can also try chanting "Om" (pronounced *Oh-m*), in which the first "Om" marks the beginning of creation (akin to the big bang in modern science). This practice is believed to build sensitivity to the outer "struck" sounds and inner "unstruck" vibrations.
- **Get closer to your belief system.** Whether you practice a particular religion or spiritual ideology, or have your own collection of truths, it's important to reconnect with your beliefs regularly. Pray, perform rituals, study texts, journal, meditate, and talk with others. What inspires you spiritually? How else can you embody your beliefs?
- **Ignite your intuition.** One way of tapping into your intuitive side is to use a tarot deck or get a tarot reading. You also may want to pick a day when you let your intuition guide you, embracing the ideas and inklings that light you up.
- **Recognize and break your addiction(s).** This can be an intense process and often requires therapy, a twelve-step program, and/or other life changes. However challenging this may be, the rewards to your health and wellness are immeasurable.

Neptune in Your Natal Chart:
Putting It to Work for You

Looking at your natal Neptune placement can help you understand how to access the healing power of Neptune. It also sheds light on where and how you can best engage your natural creativity.

Since Neptune changes zodiac signs approximately every fourteen years, I've included only eight transits, which date back to 1928 and take us to 2038.

Neptune in Virgo ♍: With the planet of dreams and mysticism in the sign of purity and devotion to spirituality, serving a cause takes a central role in life. The key word for this placement is "service."

Neptune in Libra ♎: Neptune in the sign of justice, balance, equanimity, and relationship illuminates spirituality in partnerships. The key word for this placement is "intimacy."

Neptune in Scorpio ♏: Neptune in the sign of transformation brings a deep spiritual calling to illuminate truth. The key word for this placement is "devotion."

Neptune in Sagittarius ♐: Neptune in the sign of truth and meaning brings a sense of spirituality to finding and honing your vision. The key word for this placement is "dream."

Neptune in Capricorn ♑: Neptune in the sign of practicality and business means the pragmatic can feel mystical too. The key word for this placement is "alignment."

Neptune in Aquarius ♒: Neptune in Aquarius is about dismantling practices and politics that are not humanitarian or progressive. The key word for this placement is "groundbreaking."

Neptune in Pisces ♓: Neptune in Pisces means your spiritual, artsy nature creates a sense of unity and connection with the practices you devote yourself to. The key word for this placement is "tenderhearted."

Neptune in Aries ♈: Blending spirituality and the arts with ambition, this generation will embody an esoteric understanding that we are one. The key word for this placement is "unity."

Neptune in Retrograde

Neptune's retrograde cycle lasts around five months per year. Because of his long retrograde cycle, it often goes unnoticed, unless of course he's retrograding in an important part of your chart or he's currently stationed in the sky.

However, when a Neptune transit touches an intimate part of your chart, you will feel the impact of his retrogrades. Neptune transits illuminate your highest spiritual essence but can also create a fair amount of confusion. While challenging, these periods of navigating old pain are here to guide you into a new phase of your personal journey.

Neptune Ritual: Perform a New Moon Ritual

This ritual serves to help you connect with Neptune, the planet of spirituality. In it we're going back to the basics and will be working with the new moon to set an intention for where you want to head next. We have just one chapter left in this book. You have read, grown, and integrated an incredible amount of knowledge. Now it's time to set sail in a new direction of life. A new moon ritual will support you to do just that. The new moon is a blank page, a fresh start, a moment to turn inward and consider what you want to call into your life and what you need to let go of. It's indeed a time for rest and reflection, so the perfect ritual would be in the comfort of your own home. You can do this new moon ritual either at the time of the new moon or up to two days after.

For this ritual, you'll need these items:

- Incense
- A candle
- Soothing music
- A journal
- A pen

Begin by setting up the environment. Clean and organize your space. Straightening up and getting rid of clutter sets the tone for the ceremony. I like to burn incense, light a candle, turn on soothing music, and meditate. Keep a few pieces of sacred paper and a pen on hand for writing.

As you sit at your altar, conjure a connection to the divine. Call upon a connection to the source of energy you feel supports you the most: a spiritual connection that resonates with you. Perhaps this is someone from your ancestry, a deity from your religion, or even your higher self, the part of you that's wise.

Then grab your journal and write down the things in your life you either wish to call in or are ready to release. This could be certain feelings, fears, or barriers—anything you know is not serving you. Consider what you want to call into your life. Write it out. When you're ready, put your intention into the first-person present.

The next step is to read out loud your desires—the stuff you want to call into your life now. Speaking them aloud plays a crucial role in bringing them to life. You may notice that they evoke even more emotion when spoken. That feeling is essential to manifestation.

Now that you've stated what you truly desire, sit quietly, follow your breath, and visualize your desires coming to fruition. Set the intention to stay open to these experiences entering your life, and any other growth opportunities you may need along the way. Say thank you to yourself, the divine, and your spirit.

CHAPTER 16

Pluto

Transformation and Transmutation

Holly, a mid-twenties white woman from Portland, Oregon, was getting her master's degree in clinical psychology when her ex, her first love, committed suicide. Overwhelmed by the pain of losing such an important person, but unable to process her loss, she lived with heavy guilt and remorse.

Her grief showed up as panic and urgency. She felt an enormous amount of pressure to accomplish her major life dreams... *right now!* Yet, at the same time, her extreme mood swings and other physical symptoms were impeding her progress and disrupting her overall sense of well-being.

Motivated but paralyzed, it was like she was trying to get a car out of a ditch by flooring the gas, only spinning her wheels more. She was coming apart and needed help when she came to me for coaching. She had just begun her graduate degree at a prestigious university and had an enormous amount of work ahead of her. Yet her real job was to slow down and grieve.

Since her ex's sudden death, caring for herself had felt wrong; after all, she'd failed to save one of the people she loved most. How could she take care of herself when he could no longer care for himself? We began her cosmic health journey by reframing her grieving process as a critical part of her self-care.

Little by little, she started to allow herself to experience the gut-wrenching pain of her loss. By surrendering to grief, instead of attempting to sidestep it, she could experience her heartbreak, rage, and sorrow. As she confronted this darkness, she slowly, haltingly, rediscovered herself.

Gradually, she began to reintroduce activities that made her feel good: physical exercise, dancing, art, and cultural events. She learned that grief is a lawless path, but when you stay in it, rather than try to go around it, it gives way to an important resurrection. She wasn't the same person she was before losing her loved one. However, the person she was becoming was someone she started to really love. In these and other ways, she integrated some of the intensely painful yet profoundly healing lessons of Pluto, where our tour of the planets concludes.

As the ruler of Scorpio, Pluto is the farthest from the sun. Cosmically and astrologically, he's the incarnation of darkness, both around us and inside us. As brutal as his lessons can feel, his endgame is getting us into our power, and he annihilates the status quo to force changes that we otherwise would have avoided, denied, or resisted, on behalf of our rebirth.

Inescapable Depth

Saturn defines the boundaries of our subjective consciousness—that of which we are consciously aware. Uranus represents the individualized unconscious, Neptune the collective unconscious, and Pluto the Soul itself.

—Jeffrey Wolf Green, from *Pluto Volume 1: The Evolutionary Journey of the Soul*

Pluto was the Roman god of dead souls, known as Hades to the Greeks. All mortals eventually entered his realm, referred to as Hades, Tartarus, or — only very occasionally — Erebus. The wicked were doomed to everlasting torment, and the good sent to a blessed place known as the Elysian Fields.

Pluto's power was so daunting that ancient poets rarely referred to him by name, afraid they would evoke his presence. Instead, they referred to him as Dis, which in Latin is short for *Dis Pater* and means "rich father." To downplay this fear, he became associated with Plutus, his euphemistic namesake, the Greek God of Wealth. What's notable about this is the flattery. While Pluto, as the god of the underworld, was fantastically rich, his power was so severe and tremendous that even uttering his name proved terrifying. In this new light, he still possessed fear-worthy power, but he also became closely associated with Earth's underground jewels and gems and the transformational power of rebirth.[1]

The planet Pluto consists primarily of rock and ice, and like his mythological namesake, Pluto packs a punch. Technically a dwarf planet because it's one-sixth, or 18 percent, the size of Earth's moon, Pluto is more powerful than his size suggests. He takes a no-nonsense, even ruthless approach to collective and personal transformation.

Reconciling with Loss

Pluto immerses us in our darkness, forcing us to reconcile our fear and grief, to grapple with losses that feel inescapable and all-consuming. He strips us of what is most dear and asks us to find beauty and peace as we navigate the darkness of our own depths. His invitation is for us to embrace a resurrection and rebirth, though his means are rarely gentle.

This was Holly's challenge — to delve into her traumatic grief and guilt, even dwell there, in order to heal the raw wounds in her heart and soul. By doing so, she learned so much about her strength, and how to be in pain without losing herself to it. About five years after we worked together, she reached out to let me know that she'd completed her graduate degree and made the career switch she'd long dreamed of. She'd also done some solo traveling. The trips had been cathartic. On one of them, she'd bought a bracelet to remind her that she can turn her pain into beauty and channel her strength and power into doing good in the world.

By cultivating deeper self-acceptance, including acknowledging that she's unable to "save" others from their pain, and also practicing impeccable self-care while navigating her grief, Holly learned that each day she could tip the scales toward thriving just a little bit more. This kind of unwavering perseverance and resilience is the formidable realm of Pluto. Holly's story is one of many that brings forth the intense, transformative force of this small but mighty "dwarf planet." It is here, in Pluto's domain, that we can awaken a ferocity to overcome even the most horrific circumstances. As Holly experienced, this is where we can ultimately rise and be reborn as the version of ourselves that has traveled through the pitch-black darkness inside us, only to discover a light more grounded, radiant, and real than any we've ever known.

From Death to Rebirth

Transmutation | noun

1 The action of changing or the state of being changed into another form.
1.2 *Biology, historical* The conversion or transformation of one species into another.
1.3 The supposed alchemical process of changing base metals into gold.[2]

Can we fundamentally transform? Can we be forced to handle more than we're able to and resurrect as a stronger, more resilient version of ourselves? Can we turn the "base metals" inside us into solid gold?

These are some of the questions Pluto forces us to answer. Located even farther away from the sun than Neptune, Pluto takes 247.7 years to complete its orbit around the sun. Because of this, he receives little light.

Pluto's ominous vibes also present an opportunity to settle into the trial by fire that is soul-level transformation. With Pluto as our guide, we have no choice but to look fear directly in the eye and experience it. When Pluto touches our chart, we often have to face truths we previously could not see. Here, in this challenging position, Pluto insists we see what's been hidden, however painful.

While not always pleasant, like a musical song modulating between a major key and a minor one, acclimating to our duality brings a richness to experiences that can only be accessed through darkness. Day, after all, cannot exist without night. Eager to maintain his darkness so that we may find our light, Pluto reminds us that there is a shadow side to everything, including the good. Getting comfortable with fear, and learning how to lean into our shadow, is our surest path to self-actualization, health, happiness, and liberation.

Pluto also commands us to embrace opportunities to move through stagnation, redefine our concept of ourselves, and develop meaningful and intense bonds.[3] His influence asks for refinement. While he's also deeply involved in the processes of degeneration and regeneration, his request is always the same: to metamorphose and evolve our soul. In the end, our only way forward is to metaphorically die in order to be reborn.

This transformative process is not short, simple, or straightforward. Thankfully, Pluto gives us the staying power and the determination we need to persevere. His influence becomes the push to make it through the last few miles of the marathon. Even when everything feels like it's falling apart or breaking down—and often in Pluto's presence, things do fall apart and break down—he empowers us to become our best selves while confronting the most painful, even unimaginable, circumstances.

Unlike Saturn and Mars, who give us what we can handle, Pluto serves us a whopping dose of what's beyond our capacity and stretches us to muster the resilience and grit to handle more—whether we're willing or not. This, Pluto understands, is the only way we can truly grow beyond our current limitations.

The Role of Our Shadow

According to Carl Jung, our shadow is anything that remains outside the light of our consciousness, or our conscious awareness. This can incorporate our desirable and/or our less than desirable characteristics, including the parts of us that our ego doesn't identify with. As the planet blanketed in darkness, Pluto represents our shadow.

The shadow self is often at work when we project criticism or blame onto others; have an involuntary, negative reaction or facial expression; or find damaging thoughts unconsciously creeping into our heads. This part of ourselves reveals where we may experience upheaval and power struggles. It also encompasses some of our positive qualities, yet these, too, we often fail to acknowledge.

Shadow behaviors come up during all sorts of emotions: jealousy, rage, deep disappointment, self-sabotage, narcissism, depression, etc. As excruciating as these behaviors may be, they are messengers, here to tell us something we need to hear, even when we'd rather not. They bring our attention to parts of ourselves that are informed and strengthened by our past or recurring wounds.

With Pluto, ready or not, we are given no escape route, no break, no backstage exit. There is no spiritual bypassing, no easy way to disassociate from the pain we must face. Pema Chödrön, Buddhist teacher and author of *When Things Fall Apart*, speaks to this brilliantly:

> What we're talking about is getting to know fear, becoming familiar with fear, looking it right in the eye—not as a way to solve problems but as a complete undoing of old ways of seeing, hearing, smelling, tasting, and thinking. The truth is that when we really begin to do this, we're going to be continually humbled. There's not going to be much room for the arrogance that

holding on to ideals can bring. The arrogance that inevitably does arise is going to be continually shot down by our own courage to step forward a little further. The kinds of discoveries that are made through practice have nothing to do with believing in anything. They have much more to do with having the courage to die...

Instructions on mindfulness or emptiness or working with energy all point to the same thing: being right on the spot nails us. It nails us right to the point of time and space that we are in. When we stop there and don't act out, don't repress, don't blame it on anyone else, and also don't blame it on ourselves, then we meet with an open-ended question that has no conceptual answer. We also encounter our heart.[4]

While intense, even grueling at times, this soul-level transformation is oh so necessary.

Light Isn't Everything

For sure, withstanding your shadow behavior is not fun, but ignoring your dark side only brings about the opposite effect. As Harvard psychologist Susan David notes in her book *Emotional Agility*, when you actively try not to think about something, it only becomes more potent and omnipresent. This is what psychologists call emotional leakage.[5] Disowning your shadow strengthens it.

Drowning your shadow with light doesn't work either. Don't misunderstand me here—there is immense power in positivity. I dedicated a whole chapter to techniques for conjuring a more positive outlook! Still, studies have shown that we should wield positive thinking carefully, according to our own emotional sensitivities.

In separate studies (published in 2009 and 2016), researchers found that participants who reported low self-esteem felt *even worse* after repeating or hearing positive self-statements, compared to those with low self-esteem who did not engage in affirmations.[6] The potency of positive thinking hinges on our initial self-concept: if positive self-statements fall out of the range of thoughts that we are willing to accept, we are more likely to resist them and double down on our beliefs in the counter (negative) perception.[7]

Positivity can backfire in other ways too. An overly optimistic outlook, especially one that attempts to crowd out the voice of our shadow, can lead us to overestimate our abilities,[8] underestimate difficulty, idealize future results, and engage in risky behavior.[9]

While we may yearn for light in dark times, the fact remains that light isn't everything. This is why it's so important to intimately know your shadow—it helps you keep it real. By recognizing your shadow, you can unlock your hidden beliefs, insecurities, and any pain that may be stalling your growth. From there, you can engage lines of thought and action that meet you where you are in the moment, rather than crashing and burning after indulging in optimistic overcompensation. Your ability to conjure magic hinges on your capacity to wield the power of your darkness.

WHY FEELING NEGATIVE EMOTIONS IS *GOOD* FOR YOU

Avoiding or denying natural negative emotions, like fear, sadness, or anger, stresses us out. This is the type of stress that gnaws at our well-being, as opposed to the type that boosts our resilience. However, allowing ourselves to experience our bigger, darker emotions can feel especially challenging when we've been through trauma.

If you have experienced trauma, meet yourself where it's at. Go slow, be patient, and trust. Consider doing the expressive writing activity researched by James Pennebaker that I mentioned in chapter 8 by journaling about your most difficult experience for fifteen to twenty minutes (no more than twenty minutes at a time) for four days in a row.

Expressive writing has been proven to have a long-lasting impact, increasing physical well-being and psychological well-being, and causing fewer post-traumatic intrusion symptoms. While it's normal to feel negative emotions early as you initially recall the event(s), if you have significant distress, stop and reach out for support.

Here's the prompt Pennebaker suggests:

For the next four days, I would like you to write your deepest thoughts and feelings about the most traumatic experience of your entire life or an extremely important emotional issue that has affected you. In your writing, I'd like you to really let go and explore your deepest emotions and thoughts. You might tie your topic to your relationships with others, including parents, lovers, friends, or relatives; to your past, your present, or your future; or to who you have been, who you would like to be, or who you are now. You may write about the same general issues or experiences on all days of writing or about different topics each day...Don't worry about spelling, grammar, or sentence structure. The only rule is that once you begin writing, you continue until the time is up![10]

Owning Your Shadow

Your shadow never goes away; it's an important and necessary element of your humanity. One of the best books about shadow work that I ever read was *The Dark Side of the Light Chasers* by the late Debbie Ford. Her book helped me accept the parts of myself that I had spent many years denying. After doing this work, I felt a huge release.

While shadow work isn't for the faint of heart, by doing this work we can achieve some measure of congruence between the darkness and the light inside us. It's essential to our health and wellness because it's how we come to feel a sense of wholeness.

The process begins with acknowledging the parts of yourself that you find less than desirable and bringing them into your conscious awareness. When I first engaged with shadow work, I learned that my critiques of others were actually criticisms of myself that I projected outward. It was painful admitting that, and even more agonizing shining a light on those parts of myself I didn't want to see. Yet slowly, over time, I began to make peace with the parts of myself that I'd long denied and rejected.

Here are five steps to conjure more inner harmony with your shadow:

1. **Look at what triggers you in relationships.** Pay close attention to when you feel jealousy, anger, resentment, or other challenging emotions. If you aren't feeling triggered, take a look at the qualities you admire in others. Whom do you admire and why? What we love in others are often parts of ourselves that we project outward. Take a discerning look and see what you can identify.

2. **Personify one part of you that's either triggered or projecting your light onto others.** One of my teachers calls the disowned aspects of ourselves our secret selves (yes, we have many!). Give each one your attention, name them, and get really clear on who they are. Then, choose one to work with first.

3. **Find out what she needs.** After you've identified the part of you that you want to integrate, ask her what she needs. Listen deeply and hear what she's craving. What is your secret self asking of you? What does she need that your day-to-day life doesn't let her experience? Set an intention that honors her needs, and write it out affirmatively in the first person. Then read it out loud, allowing it to sink into your conscious and unconscious mind.

4. **Take action.** Once you discover what the disowned aspect of yourself is asking for, offer her what she's craving. For example, perhaps she craves frivolity, and this manifests as overeating

sugar, particularly ice cream. But what if you gave her a playdate and let her embrace the joy of play without needing to be so measured or as intentional as daily life requires?

5. **Learn the art of distress tolerance.** Being okay with not being okay takes practice. That's ultimately what resilience is: to face life exactly as it is, and rise anyway. It's an act of fully accepting things as they are while simultaneously responding to them with strength. Hope, then, is not about negating but rather accepting what is—and still finding ways to incrementally make things better. The more you can lean into and be with fear and discomfort, the more you can accept their presence and use them to your advantage. The more you embrace the inner vulnerability required to see yourself with radical honesty, the quicker you can find true harmony within yourself and in your relationships with others. I encourage you to go inward with a flashlight and bring the unconscious to the surface.

Navigating Death, Dying, and Loss

As the planet that rules Scorpio, and the sign of death and rebirth, depth and power, Pluto teaches us about grief and many forms of loss, including fertility struggles and miscarriages.

On top of the pain and grief that fertility issues cause, many women end up navigating their pain alone and largely in silence. Since miscarriages are fairly common, the depth and breadth of the grief they can cause is too often ignored or overlooked. At the same time, fertility struggles remain, even now, a sort of taboo topic. While there's increasing openness about fertility struggles in mass media, many of my clients have grieved privately, only confessing their enduring sadness and shame years later. It's heartbreaking grief that many ultimately have to live with and a journey that's substantially more intense for parents who have lost a child.

While the pain of these losses is undeniably harsh and long-lasting, we can ultimately choose to heal, and in so doing, we gain a firm grasp of the truth of who we are and what and who truly matters to us. However, there's no denying that this healing process is harrowing and not one we can rush through. Even if we are fortunate enough to finally have a healthy child, we can't nullify the grief of the previous pregnancies or the child we lost.

Yet eventually, and with tremendous support throughout, we can embody the darkness of our grief while also receiving the light, love, and joy that comes into our lives. As Holly did, we can allow ourselves to be broken and whole at the same time; we can be simultaneously grateful and grief-stricken. In her email to me years later, she shared that she had been able to finally "find joy and make room for struggle." This is relevant for all forms of loss, including letting go of an identity and more. That is what Pluto asks us to do: to embrace and embody the inherent duality inside us.

With Pluto as our guide, we can integrate these polarities and let them transform us at the most profound and essential level. This is the opportunity for transmutation that is written into Pluto's cosmic mission.

Stepping into Our Power

Transformation is an inherent part of stepping into our power, yet so often we fear the power we have. Why? Because we rise and fall; we shine and dim. This is what cyclical living is about: understanding that things come together for a while and then change. Our goal, then, is to develop the resilience to be with this process, to navigate it *without* checking out or running from pain, fear, or discomfort. Instead, we can lean into our challenging and dark emotions, and grow stronger and more resilient from what they teach us. From our darkness, we resurrect.

Like Earth, rotating on its axis at a tilt and receiving different amounts of sunlight based on where it is relative to the sun, we, too, have moments of exaltation and moments of annihilation. This is what it means to be human. While Pluto can have scary connotations, he is here to teach us to live in harmony with the death-and-rebirth cycle we can't escape. With Pluto, the loss we navigate always has a purpose; it's our initiation into rebirth.

Pluto in Your Natal Chart: Putting It to Work for You

With Pluto spending extended periods of time in each sign, his placement in your chart is a generational one. Like Neptune, I listed Pluto through the signs for a limited number of years: 1939 to 2043.

> **Pluto in Leo ♌:** Pluto in Leo issues a call to reclaim the inner child and reimagine your relationship to joy, pleasure, and freedom. Developing self-reliance, confidence, and independence is key.
>
> **Pluto in Virgo ♍:** Pluto in Virgo seeks a disruption to the status quo around health, the environment, and food. Your task includes bringing a deeper sense of spirituality to your day-to-day life, routine, and health habits by identifying a purpose that guides your existence.
>
> **Pluto in Libra ♎:** Pluto in Libra issues a call to redefine your relationships, bringing the self into partnerships, integrating the "me" in "we." Your focus is on fairness, justice, and balance.
>
> **Pluto in Scorpio ♏:** Pluto in Scorpio asks you to face shadows around the most quintessential taboos of life: sex, death, finances, and other power dynamics. Focus on embodiment and cultivate a regenerative, nonexploitative lifestyle.
>
> **Pluto in Sagittarius ♐:** Pluto in Sagittarius issues a call to find a personal philosophy that works for you. Step out of the dogma of religion and into the essence of personal freedom. Focus on developing a diverse community, perhaps leveraging social media.

Pluto in Capricorn ♑: Pluto in Capricorn focuses on disassembling the patriarchy, reconciling the lost art of feminine practices, dismantling racism, and standing up to oppression.

Pluto in Aquarius ♒: Pluto in Aquarius puts an emphasis on learning how to collectively share resources and work toward realizing a world where everyone can thrive with equal access to Earth's resources.

Pluto in Retrograde

Pluto retrogrades for up to six months and only by a couple of degrees. As a result, his retrogrades are typically felt collectively more than personally.

When a Pluto transit touches an intimate part of your chart, though, you will feel the impact of his retrograde. However challenging, these periods of navigating pain are here to guide you into a new phase of life, and your personal rebirth. I have observed with Pluto transits that there's usually an initial introduction to the cosmic curriculum that this transit brings, which can feel shocking; afterward, the intensity of the transit stabilizes. Pluto's retrograde cycle is an opportunity to integrate these teachings and find power in your emerging strength.

Pluto Ritual: Embracing Your Resurrection

Having endured grief and loss, we often forgo the most important practice for rebirth: giving ourselves the tender loving care we routinely give to others. Now, as you reemerge as more radiant and empowered, it's essential for you to view radical self-care as what it is: the foundation of your cosmic health and the healing magic it awakens. The simple truth is, neither you nor I can conjure our best and brightest healing—in our health, our lives, our hearts, or our souls—from a place of perpetual depletion.

This ritual, which begins with a short meditation, will guide you into an enduring commitment to your own tender loving care. Return to this ritual as often as you like. It is here, in this place of sacred self-nurturing, that your rebirth and resurrection take root.

Radical Self-Care Meditation

Before beginning, make sure to have a journal and pen or pencil nearby.

Sit quietly and tune in to your higher self. Think of your higher self as your observer, she who witnesses you without feeding into drama or amplifying emotion. This part of you is wise, loving, and compassionate. Where you see flaws, she sees beauty. Where you see wounds, she sees strength and renewal. She is your inner phoenix, forever supporting your rise from the proverbial ashes. Trust her, unconditionally and always.

Settling into this connection, meditate for five to ten minutes, focusing on your breath as the air comes in and goes out. Breathe deeply, allowing the air to descend into the base of your belly, which calms your nervous system and supports a healthy detachment from your emotions.

Once you can observe your life from a distance, as if you were watching yourself from ten thousand feet above, tune in and ask yourself, *What does radical self-care look like for me in this moment?*

If you were to create an action plan for your cosmic health and self-care, what would you tend to first? Where in your body, life, or emotions do you *know* you need to experience more peace? What would feel most nourishing and soothing at this time?

Once you get a sense of your needs, write down whatever comes to mind. It might be a long walk, less socializing, a therapy session, or a massage. Often little changes make the biggest difference in our health: eating more vegetables, decreasing sugar or alcohol intake, breathing deeply, journaling, drinking more water, taking vitamins, adding regular cardiovascular activity. These are the small but mighty action steps that bring us back to center.

Now that you've gained more clarity on the kind of self-care you most need, you are ready for your resurrection ritual.

Resurrection Ritual

You will need a printed copy of your astrological chart, a picture of you as a child, and a quiet spot in which to conduct your ritual.

Begin by looking at your astrological chart. Consider the zodiac signs, the different planets, as well as the dominant elements (earth, air, fire, water) and modes (cardinal, fixed, mutable) in your chart. Ask yourself, *What is the truest expression of my chart? What does this chart desire for me? What kind of elevation or transformation is my chart calling me toward?*

In a loving voice, say out loud whatever comes to you.

Next, ask yourself, *What kind of self-care will best support me right now?*

Commit to this one act of self-care that supports and nourishes your soul.

Once you've determined the action step you will take today, or in the next twenty-four hours, ask for divine support and guidance throughout your healing journey.

Now, look at the picture of you as a child. Study it.

Meditate on your strengths. Feel wholehearted appreciation for all that you have learned and experienced.

Ask yourself, *What am I most grateful for?* In a loving voice, say out loud whatever comes to you. (Take as long as need.)

When you feel complete, put your hands on your heart. Tenderly connect with your younger self, you as a child, and offer yourself loving-kindness.

Finally, look at your chart and the picture of you again..

Whisper the words "Thank you."

Sometimes the most powerful transformation comes from taking the next step or even the next breath. Resilience means accepting where you are now while also moving toward your most radiant and abundant cosmic health.

Conclusion

We began with Chaos and her unfathomable darkness.

We conclude with Circe and her bewitching magic.

Skilled at turning lustful drunkards into actual swine, Circe conjured spells potent enough to protect her son from the mighty goddess Athena, and with practice and perseverance, her sorcery grew legendary.

Aware of her power as well as her vulnerabilities, Circe eventually betrayed the eternal exile imposed upon her by Zeus and descended deep into the sea. There, immersed in a terrible, undefinable darkness, she sought out the fearsome beast Trygon. Drawing strength from her purpose, passion, and maternal love, she reached out in sacrifice, prepared to accept the poison that seemed her ultimate fate. To protect her son from Athena, she would soon live in eternal pain. Yet seeking her punishment in the watery depths around her, she found nothing.

"That is enough," Trygon declared.

Already aligned with her true purpose, Circe, who had faced many fears and had known a great deal of pain and punishment—a love-starved childhood followed by eternal exile and abuse at the hands of mortal men—was spared this brutal poison. Unlike her sorcerer brother and the many gods who had tried and failed before her, only she was permitted to slice off Trygon's tail. (It contained a poison even the gods were not immune to and had long been coveted by men and gods as a result.) Humbled by gratitude, Circe quietly returned to the island of her exile and gave the formidable weapon to her son to use in self-defense during his first solo voyage.

This story, written by Madeline Miller,[1] portrays Circe's courage, conviction, and magic, but of course none of these qualities are new. You may not have known it then, but you encountered magic in the first pages of this book, in the initial moment of this journey and many others, amidst the all-consuming darkness of your own chaos.

When we have felt our weakest, most disoriented, and most vulnerable, we are already beginning to conjure and transform. Like each night, when in total darkness Earth rotates to make way for daybreak; like each lunar cycle, when pitch-blackness ushers us into the full moon's radiance; like the seasons and the zodiac, which illuminate the many facets of our most radiant well-being, within you and me there is an abundance of magic.

Magic is the act of creation through intention and will, in communion with forces outside ourselves. Fueled by love, it offers us incredible freedom, as its very essence is a manifestation of equal opportunity. You do not have to know magic's inner workings to wield it for self-development and willful creation. You do not need to defer to any single source or higher power. Your magic—indeed all magic—is simultaneously omnipresent and deeply personal.

Circe worked tirelessly at cultivating her sorcery, gathering herbs and investing hours that turned into weeks, then years, harnessing each herb's, potion's, and spell's true power. She also immersed herself in the natural world, meandering through deep forests and befriending the wild and mighty creatures in her midst. Perhaps most notable of all, throughout her many trials and tribulations, she conjured inside herself, even in the hardest of times, the focused intention to cultivate more personal power and love, always nurturing her truest, deepest essence.

This, in many ways, is where your magic must now take root and blossom—as a seedling inside you that bolsters your focused intention to create and receive your own brand of cosmic health. While cosmic health amplifies magic, it is derived from magic too. We see this play out in Circe, who herself only became the creatrix she was meant to be once she decided to inhabit her innate inclinations.

You, too, are discovering that seedling inside you. You, too, are learning to sway with the rhythms within and around you, as well as the planets and their energetic interactions with your natal chart and your life. You, too, are deciding to pursue and refine your healing power.

The seemingly esoteric connections we made early in this book are perhaps just now beginning to make real sense. We are stardust; we are unavoidably interconnected. The cosmos that surrounds us affects us from our skin's surface straight through to our soul, emotions, mindset, desires, and self-expression. The cycles that control the sun and the moon also influence our biology. We embody ideas and emotions that radiate through our physical bodies, our lives, and those around us.

We are interconnected, in every way, on every level. We are the physical and spiritual manifestations of the concept of "both/and." We have real science — and real magic too.

This constant flow of data and rhythm — from our heart, soul, and body, from the planets as they interact with our natal chart and cosmic curriculum, from our thoughts and emotions as they manifest in the body and ripple throughout our lives — is at the core of cosmic health. The conditions we experience, externally and internally, are forever changing. Our aim now, as always, is to develop the spiritual muscle to rise and conjure, as Circe did, again and again. Rather than attaching ourselves to fixed definitions of health, wellness, success, happiness, or even love, we must continuously fortify our ability to flex with the changing seasons of our soul, mind, body, and environs, to heal ourselves on every level by learning to flow through labor and rest, giving and receiving.

With time and practice, we can use our magic, the healing magic of cosmic health, to dance with the undulations inside and around us. We can continue to fine-tune ourselves according to the rhythms of the seasons, heeding our basic nature and cosmic curriculum, and responding as the planets touch our natal chart, our minds, our emotions, and our lives. With the tenets of cosmic health in our spiritual tool kit, we, like Circe, can ebb and flow with ever-changing conditions. We are the enchantresses of the health we desire.

In the end, Circe's grandest accomplishment wasn't securing Trygon's tail. It was facing each of her most formidable foes — her own father, Helios, god of the sun, and Athena, goddess of wisdom and war. In spite of what protocol mandated, Circe didn't grovel or beg from either of these mighty divinities. Instead, she stood firmly and spoke her truth. While only a demigod herself, Circe used her intellect, courage, and magic to command respect from those who felt inclined to give her none. That sense of self, and that commitment to self-love too, is embedded in your healing evolution.

It should be noted that Circe never stopped conjuring the seemingly impossible. Against all odds, she regained her freedom. No longer exiled, she found lasting love and traveled the world, collecting exotic and powerful herbs as she went. She also took Penelope, wife of the late Odysseus, who had once been Circe's illicit lover, as her apprentice. Penelope then discovered the depth and breadth of her own magic.

Let us follow Circe's lead and share cosmic health with the women around us. As your healing capacities grow, lead another toward hers.

So much in our world needs healing. We must harness our power to heal ourselves, then others, and, in turn, our world. It is time, and you are far more powerful than you know.

Come, conjure with me, and heal.

My love always,
Jenn

Acknowledgments

Positive psychology teaches us to cultivate our strengths, develop our resilience, and feel our emotions fully, especially gratitude! Writing a book is an amazing privilege full of many twists and turns. I am sincerely humbled and amazed by how many hands are involved in making a book possible.

To my agent, Wendy Sherman, who believed in this book from the minute I mentioned it. You stood by me the whole way, offering advice at critical times and shepherding this project along as needed. You are the best! I am sincerely grateful for all of your support. Thank you.

Marisa Vigilante, your encouragement, enthusiasm, and insight made working with you a highlight of my career. I am most grateful to you for making *Cosmic Health* possible. To Ian Strauss, your empathy, compassion, and support helped birth this book. You were gracious every step of the way. Thank you! To Dianna Stirpe, your copy edits were astute and precise. You elevated this project. I am most grateful. Jessica Chun and Juliana Horbachevsky, thank you for your care with public relations and marketing. To the whole Little, Brown Spark team from production to design, especially Ben Allen and Karen Landry—you brought my vision to life. I am thrilled and grateful.

To my family, all of you: Mom, Dad, Diane, Phil, John, Toula, Michele, Sophia, Annabella, Olivia, I love you so much. Thank you for championing my journey. Doug Bandes, you have taught me the meaning of grit, resilience, and humility. Thank you for always believing in me. To both the Bandes + Golden families, thank you for being a part of my life.

My teachers and mentors, without whom my thinking on this topic wouldn't be possible: Maria Sirois, Dr. Tal Ben-Shahar, Debra Silverman, Rebecca Gordon, Debbie Lefay, Freedom Cole, Naina Marballi, Dr. Jeffrey Migdow, Melanie Smith, and the many others who have guided me along the way. Thank you. And extra thanks to Maria, for helping me through the proposal process and the initial phases of writing this book.

I stand upon the shoulders of giants. Astrology when done well is as academic as it is spiritual. I am sincerely grateful to the generations of astrologers who have come before me and those who are still working tirelessly to elevate this craft and field. Thank you.

To everyone who collaborated with me on this book, you made it possible. Marisol Dahl, your contributions from the very first thought were a remarkable gift. Your support with research and developing ideas shaped the book immensely. Andrea Hannah, your supportive ear, investigative mind, and sensibilities as a writer helped me more than you know. Wyndham Wood, you are a friend and a mentor with a knack for avoiding the weeds and getting to the heart of how to structure a book and tell a story well. You taught me so much. I am most grateful. Thank you! Richelle Fredson, you mentored me, believed in me, gave me critical feedback, and elevated me every step along the way.

Allie Mason, you have been an integral part of my creative process for a very long time. Thank you for all of your support and understanding of the immense brainpower it took to write this book while I took so much time away from my business to get it done. Yael Passerelli, Toi Smith, and June Foret, you helped hold down my business while I gave my all to this project, and you too are a critical part of the team that helped birth this book.

Gemini Brett, your support as a colleague and your mastery of your skill set are deeply appreciated and admired. To my beta readers at

Acknowledgments

Quiethouse Editing, your feedback was to the point and spot-on, and it strengthened the material.

Kristen Sbrogna, you've been along for the ride with me since that fated day I met Debbie in Lake Tahoe. Without your friendship, I wouldn't be here. I am also sincerely so lucky that you, my dear friend, also hold both an MFA and a PhD. I never expected you to offer me and this book so much of your time and expertise. Thank you for reading it (multiple times) and for providing me very thoughtful feedback and edits along the way. I am so grateful. Nitika Chopra, you have championed my work for years and held me through the roughest moments of this creative process. I love you. Mimi Klein, where do I even start?! Your support has been so crucial, not just to this book but to my life in general. A million thanks. Dana Weissman, you were so gracious with all of my proofreads. Thank you for your friendship and kindness.

Alison Leipzig, Michelle Garside, and Hannah Coward of Soul Camp Creative, your design direction and illustrations showed me possibilities I didn't even consider. Thank you for your patience with me as I sometimes took an extra-long time responding to emails. You did a fantastic job.

Nicole Jardim and Jenny Sansouci, what better way to slug through the book-writing process than with you two whip-smart, newly minted authors by my side? Doing this together made being a rookie all the better.

To Jen, Karen, Sandy, Abby, and Kristin, you supported me all those years ago through my cancer journey and especially the last six months as I finished this book. Without you, I couldn't have done any of this. Thank you.

Natalie Berthold, Emily Pitcher, Ginni Guiton, and Kathleen Hall, you held me through some of the hardest parts of this process. I am forever grateful.

Kate Northrup, Sarah Jenks, Eliza Reynolds, Nisha Moodley, Briana Borten, Kavita Patel, Grace Smith, Katie Den Ouden, Sarah Adler, Alex Jamieson, Bex Boruki, Colette Baron Reid, and Gina DeVee, you are the most amazing colleagues. Thank you for championing me and helping me in all the ways you have.

To all my friends, you make life a little extra-*cosmic*, and I wouldn't want to do it any other way.

Most importantly, to my clients who have trusted me as their coach and astrologer—an extremely special role indeed—thank you. Without you, this book would not be possible, especially the clients who have allowed me to capture their stories in this book. I am incredibly grateful.

To everyone who bought or read *Cosmic Health*, may you all unlock your healing magic as you step into your resilience. Remember, your chaos is a window to more joy and meaning. Thank you.

To the sky, I will forever be your student with full humility.

Author's Note on Sources and Presentation

Throughout this book, I share stories of some of the many incredible women I'm fortunate to coach. While all of these inspiring women agreed to have their stories told in this book, to protect their privacy I've changed their names and personal details. Three of the stories shared are composites of multiple clients.

Where useful, I have referenced scientific research. Scientific findings are sometimes used, even misused, as justifications for extreme political and social views. Absolutely none of the science I refer to in this book suggests or is intended to express any underlying assumptions or viewpoints. My interest is strictly in the science itself and how it can serve us—all of us—to achieve more radiant cosmic health.

This book is about your cosmic health and how it's affected by your personal natal chart; that is to say, this is not a collective astrology book. The transpersonal planets—Uranus, Neptune, and Pluto—often also have a broader cultural impact. For our purposes, they are largely discussed through a more personal cosmic health.

Astrology is the science and art of understanding corollaries. This book looks at the relationship between astrology and the modern sciences of wellness, healing, and happiness. This is not a medical astrology book, and I am not a medical astrologer. While there are aspects of this book that lean into the wisdom of medical astrology, cosmic health does not rely on, or even necessitate, the application of medical astrology.

While this book will help you to gain a deeper understanding of your own chart and its significance in your life and cosmic health, it does not attempt to train anyone to become an astrologer. Astrology is an ancient practice that takes years to master. In the appendix of this book I list astrologers and organizations that I either have studied with or am a member of for anyone who wishes to study it in more depth.

Finally, the origins of magic reach back centuries. The word *magic* derives from the old Persian *maguš* and its root *magh*, meaning "be able." Although astrology and astrological magic come from very different lineages, as a white woman, it is important to acknowledge the many Indigenous peoples who have long worked with the Earth's cycles and maintained traditions distinctly theirs, despite a longstanding history of genocide and forced removal. I respectfully acknowledge the land I live and work on as the unceded land of the Mohicans.

Please come to JenniferRacioppi.com/resources and download the ebook that accompanies *Cosmic Health*!

Appendix A

Astrologers and Astrology Organizations for Continued Learning

Debra Silverman: debrasilvermanastrology.com

NCGR, National Council for Geocosmic Research: geocosmic.org

OPA, the Organization for Professional Astrology: opaastrology.org

ISAR, International Society for Astrological Research: isarastrology.org

Rebecca Gordon: rebeccagordonastrology.com

Gemini Brett: geminibrett.com

Astrology Books

The Only Way to Learn Astrology, volumes 1 and 2, by Marion D. March and Joan McEvers

Mysteries of the Dark Moon: The Healing Power of the Dark Goddess by Demetra George

Your Body and the Stars: The Zodiac as Your Wellness Guide by Stephanie Marango and Rebecca Gordon

The Twelve Houses: Exploring the Houses of the Horoscope by Howard Sasportas

The Missing Element: Inspiring Compassion for the Human Condition by Debra Silverman

New Moon Astrology: The Secret of Astrological Timing to Make All Your Dreams Come True by Jan Spiller

Appendix B

Infographic: Decoding Your Natal Chart

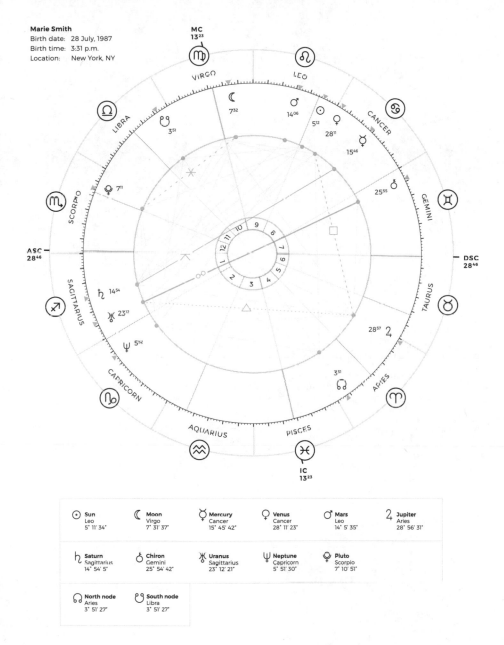

Marie Smith
Birth date: 28 July, 1987
Birth time: 3:31 p.m.
Location: New York, NY

☉ Sun	☽ Moon	☿ Mercury	♀ Venus	♂ Mars	♃ Jupiter
Leo	Virgo	Cancer	Cancer	Leo	Aries
5° 11' 34"	7° 31' 37"	15° 45' 42"	28° 11' 23"	14° 5' 35"	28° 56' 31"

♄ Saturn	⚷ Chiron	♅ Uranus	♆ Neptune	♇ Pluto	
Sagittarius	Gemini	Sagittarius	Capricorn	Scorpio	
14° 54' 5"	25° 54' 42"	23° 12' 21"	5° 51' 30"	7° 10' 51"	

☊ North node	☋ South node
Aries	Libra
3° 51' 27"	3° 51' 27"

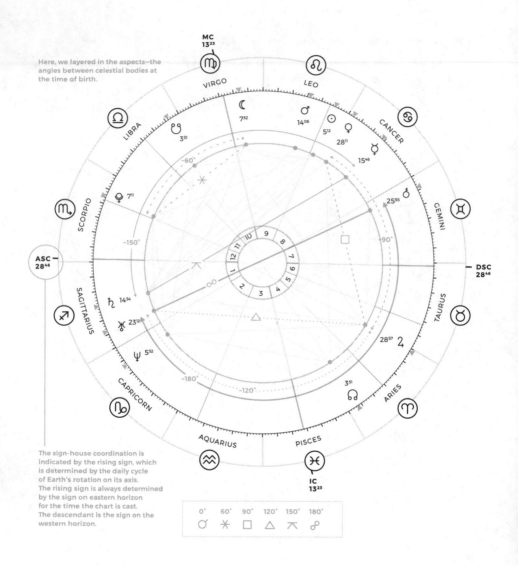

Here, we layered in the aspects—the angles between celestial bodies at the time of birth.

The sign-house coordination is indicated by the rising sign, which is determined by the daily cycle of Earth's rotation on its axis. The rising sign is always determined by the sign on eastern horizon for the time the chart is cast. The descendant is the sign on the western horizon.

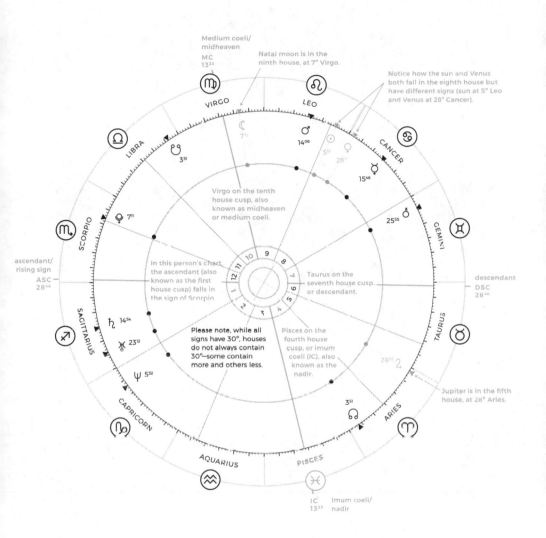

Medium coeli/
midheaven
MC
13²³

Natal moon is in the
ninth house, at 7° Virgo.

Notice how the sun and Venus
both fall in the eighth house but
have different signs (sun at 5° Leo
and Venus at 28° Cancer).

VIRGO

LEO

CANCER

LIBRA

GEMINI

Virgo on the tenth
house cusp, also
known as midheaven
or medium coeli.

SCORPIO

ascendant/
rising sign
ASC
28⁴⁶

In this person's chart,
the ascendant (also
known as the first
house cusp) falls in
the sign of Scorpio.

Taurus on the
seventh house cusp,
or descendant.

descendant
DSC
28⁴⁶

SAGITTARIUS

TAURUS

Please note, while all
signs have 30°, houses
do not always contain
30°—some contain
more and others less.

Pisces on the
fourth house
cusp, or imum
coeli (IC), also
known as the
nadir.

Jupiter is in the fifth
house, at 28° Aries.

CAPRICORN

ARIES

AQUARIUS

PISCES

IC
13²³

Imum coeli/
nadir

Notes

Preface

1. Edith Hamilton, *Mythology: Timeless Tales of Gods and Heroes* (New York: Black Dog & Leventhal, 2017).

Introduction

1. National Wellness Institute, "Definition of Wellness: The Six Dimensions of Wellness," accessed May 13, 2020, https://nationalwellness.org/resources/six -dimensions-of-wellness.
2. Purely to facilitate the discussion necessitated by each of these planets, I use the gender—"she" or "he"—commonly assigned to each planet. But please note the pronouns are not definitive. Astrology originated at a time when traditional gender roles were the only option. We certainly have come a long way.

Chapter 1: The Five Principles of Cosmic Health

1. Phoebe Wyss, *Inside the Cosmic Mind: Archetypal Astrology and the New Cosmology* (Edinburgh, UK: Floris Books, 2014).
2. Angela Duckworth, *Grit: The Power of Passion and Perseverance* (New York: Scribner, 2016); and Angela Duckworth, "What Is Grit?" FAQ, accessed May 13, 2020, https:// angeladuckworth.com/qa/#faq-125.
3. Jim Collins, "Genius of the And," accessed May 13, 2020, https://www.jimcollins .com/concepts/genius-of-the-and.html.
4. Barbara Ehrenreich and Deidre English, *Witches, Midwives, and Nurses: A History of Women Healers* (New York: Feminist Press at CUNY, 2010).

Chapter 2: Astrology and Health

1. Liz Greene, *Jung's Studies in Astrology: Prophecy, Magic, and the Qualities of Time* (London and New York: Routledge, 2018).
2. C. G. Jung, *Jung on Astrology*, eds. Safron Rossi and Keiron Le Grice (New York: Routledge, 2017).
3. Richard Tarnas, *Cosmos and Psyche: Intimations of a New World View* (New York: Viking, 2006). For more on this topic, also check out Keiron Le Grice, "Jung on Synchronicity and the Mechanism for Astrology," interview by Chris Brennan, *The*

Astrology Podcast, episode 148, March 16, 2018, https://theastrologypodcast.com /2018/03/16/jung-on-synchronicity-and-the-mechanism-for-astrology/.

4. Simon Worrall, "How 40,000 Tons of Cosmic Dust Falling to Earth Affects You and Me," *National Geographic*, January 28, 2015, https://news.nationalgeographic .com/2015/01/150128-big-bang-universe-supernova-astrophysics-health-space -ngbooktalk/.

5. Gemini Brett, "The Very Real Astronomy of Tropical Astrology," YouTube video, 2:49:50, posted April 16, 2019, https://www.youtube.com/watch?v=UMsrA1JdSYE.

6. Harry F. Darling, *Essentials of Medical Astrology* (Tempe, AZ: American Federation of Astrologers, 1981).

Chapter 3: Living in Sync with Lunar Cycles

1. University of Jefferson Myra Brind Center of Integrative Medicine, "How Emotional Processes Affect Physical Health and Well Being," Topics in Integrative Medicine, https://jdc.jefferson.edu/jmbcim/13/.

2. Rosemarie Kobau et al., "Mental Health Promotion in Public Health: Perspectives and Strategies from Positive Psychology," *American Journal of Public Health* 101, no. 8 (2011): e1–e9.

3. Florian Raible, Hiroki Takekata, and Kristin Tessmar-Raible, "An Overview of Monthly Rhythms and Clocks," *Frontiers in Neurology* 8 (2017): 189; and Gabriele Andreatta and Kristin Tessmar-Raible, "The Still Dark Side of the Moon: Molecular Mechanisms of Lunar-Controlled Rhythms and Clocks," *Journal of Molecular Biology* 432, no. 12 (2020): 3525–46.

4. Raible, Takekata, and Tessmar-Raible, "An Overview of Monthly Rhythms and Clocks," 189.

5. Nicole Jardim, *Fix Your Period: Six Weeks to Banish Bloating, Conquer Cramps, Manage Moodiness, and Ignite Lasting Hormonal Balance* (New York: HarperCollins, 2020).

6. Sandra J. Kuhlman, L. Michon Craig, and Jeanne F. Duffy, "Introduction to Chronobiology," *Cold Spring Harbor Perspectives in Biology* 10, no. 9 (2018): a033613.

Chapter 4: Living in Sync with Solar Cycles

1. Gavin W. Lambert et al., "Effect of Sunlight and Season on Serotonin Turnover in the Brain," *The Lancet* 360, no. 9348 (2002): 1840–42, https://www.thelancet.com /journals/lancet/article/PIIS0140-6736(02)11737-5/fulltext.

2. Richard J. Wurtman and Judith J. Wurtman, "Brain Serotonin, Carbohydrate-Craving, Obesity, and Depression," *Obesity Research* 3, suppl. 4 (1995): 477–80S.

3. Alfred J. Lewy et al., "The Circadian Basis for Winter Depression," *PNAS* 103, no. 19 (2006): 7414–19.

4. Michael Terman et al., "Controlled Trial of Naturalistic Dawn Simulation and Negative Air Ionization for Seasonal Affective Disorder," *American Journal of Psychiatry* 163, no. 12 (2006): 2126–33; and Konstantin V. Danilenko and Iana A. Ivanova, "Dawn Simulation vs. Bright Light in Seasonal Affective Disorder: Treatment Effects and Subjective Preference," *Journal of Affective Disorders* 180 (2015): 87–89.

5. Rachel Leproult et al., "Transition from Dim to Bright Light in the Morning Induces an Immediate Elevation of Cortisol Levels," *Journal of Clinical Endocrinology and Metabolism* 86, no. 1 (2001): 151–57.

6. Madeline Kennedy, "Morning Daylight Exposure Tied to a Good Night's Sleep," Reuters, May 18, 2017, https://www.reuters.com/article/us-health-sleep-daylight/morning-daylight-exposure-tied-to-a-good-nights-sleep-idUSKCN18E23E.

7. Northwestern University, "Bright Light Alters Metabolism," *Science Daily*, May 18, 2016, https://www.sciencedaily.com/releases/2016/05/160518141416.htm.

8. John and Peter Filbey, *Astrology for Astrologers: An Introduction to the Astronomical Basis for Modern Astrology* (Willingborough, Northamptonshire: The Aquarian Press, 1984).

Chapter 5: The Moon Sign: Learning How to Self-Nuture

1. OWN, "Dr. Brené Brown on Joy: It's Terrifying | SuperSoul Sunday | Oprah Winfrey Network," YouTube video, 5:58, posted March 17, 2013, https://www.youtube.com/watch?v=RKV0BWSPfOw&feature.

2. Christian G, "Tal Ben-Shahar—Permission to Be Human," YouTube video, 19:17, posted August 29, 2013, https://www.youtube.com/watch?v=1hFyjy9P5lg&.

3. Resmaa Menakem, *My Grandmother's Hands: Racialized Trauma and the Pathway to Mending Our Hearts and Bodies* (Las Vegas, NV: Central Recovery Press, 2017).

4. J. Lee Lehman, Ph.D., *Classical Astrology for Modern Living: From Ptolemy to Psychology & Back Again* (Atglen, PA: Whitford Press, 1996).

Chapter 6: The Sun Sign: Be Who You Are

1. David Schnarch, *Intimacy and Desire: Awaken the Passion in Your Relationship* (New York: Beaufort Books, 2009).

2. Donna Hicks, *Dignity: The Essential Role It Plays in Resolving Conflict* (New Haven, CT: Yale Univ. Press, 2011).

3. Meggan Watterson, *Reveal: A Sacred Manual for Getting Spiritually Naked* (Carlsbad, CA: Hay House, 2013).

4. Stephanie Marango and Rebecca Gordon, *Your Body and the Stars: The Zodiac as Your Wellness* (New York: Atria, 2016).

Chapter 7: The Rising Sign: Own Your Awesome

1. Catherine P. Cook-Cottone, "Incorporating Positive Body Image into the Treatment of Eating Disorders: A Model for Attunement and Mindful Self-Care," *Body Image* 14 (2015): 158–67.

2. Sonja Lyubomirsky, Laura King, and Ed Diener, "The Benefits of Frequent Positive Affect: Does Happiness Lead to Success?" *Psychological Bulletin* 131, no. 6 (2005): 803–55, http://www.apa.org/pubs/journals/releases/bul-1316803.pdf.

3. Positive Psychology Center, "Perma Theory of Well-Being and Perma Workshops," School of Arts and Sciences, University of Pennsylvania, accessed July 14, 2020, https://ppc.sas.upenn.edu/learn-more/perma-theory-well-being-and-perma-workshops.

Chapter 8: Mercury: Can You Really Have What You Want?

1. Edith Hamilton, *Mythology* (New York: Little, Brown, 1976).
2. Poptech, "Ellen Langer: Mindfulness Over Matter," YouTube video, 22:20, posted November 5, 2013, https://www.youtube.com/watch?v=4XQUJR4uIGM. Also check out her book about how mindset influences health outcomes, based on her findings with the Counterclockwise study: Ellen J. Langer, *Counterclockwise: Mindful Health and the Power of Possibility* (New York: Ballantine Books, 2009).
3. Ellen J. Langer, *Counterclockwise: Mindful Health and the Power of Possibility* (New York: Ballantine Books, 2009).
4. Association for Psychological Science, "Do You Really Need Those Eyeglasses?" April 2, 2010, https://www.psychologicalscience.org/news/were-only-human/do-you-really-need-those-eyeglasses.html.
5. Chanmo Park et al., "Blood Sugar Level Follows Perceived Time Rather than Actual Time in People with Type 2 Diabetes," *PNAS* 113, no. 29 (2016): 8168–70.
6. Bruce Grierson, "What If Age Is Nothing but a Mind-Set?" *New York Times Magazine,* Health Issue, October 22, 2015, https://www.nytimes.com/2014/10/26/magazine/what-if-age-is-nothing-but-a-mind-set.html.
7. Karen A. Baikie and Kay Wilhelm, "Emotional and Physical Health Benefits of Expressive Writing," *Advances in Psychiatric Treatment* 11, no. 5 (2005): 338–46, https://www.americansforthearts.org/sites/default/files/338full.pdf.
8. Ellen J. Langer, "The Third Metric for Success," blog at ellenlanger.com, 2009, https://www.ellenlanger.com/blog/171/the-third-metric-for-success.

Chapter 9: Venus: Beauty, Love, and Body—Harnessing Your Power

1. Alia J. Crum, Peter Salovey, and Shawn Achor, "Rethinking Stress: The Role of Mindsets in Determining the Stress Response," *Journal of Personality and Social Psychology* 104, no. 4 (2013): 716–33.
2. Eva Pool et al., "Stress Increases Cue-Triggered 'Wanting' for Sweet Reward in Humans," *Journal of Experimental Psychology* 41, no. 2 (2015): 128–36, https://www.apa.org/pubs/journals/releases/xan-0000052.pdf.
3. Kara Mayer Robinson, "10 Surprising Health Benefits of Sex," WebMD, last modified October 24, 2013, https://www.webmd.com/sex-relationships/guide/sex-and-health#1.

Chapter 10: Mars: Planet of Action and Motivation

1. John T. Ratey, *Spark: The Revolutionary New Science of Exercise and the Brain* (New York: Little, Brown Spark, 2008).
2. TEDx Talks, "Run, Jump, Learn! How Exercise Can Transform Our Schools: John J. Ratey, MD, at TEDxManhattanBeach," YouTube video, 10:43, posted November 18, 2012, https://youtu.be/hBSVZdTQmDs.
3. Duke Today Staff, "Study: Exercise Has Long-Lasting Effect on Depression," Duke University, September 22, 2000, https://today.duke.edu/2000/09/exercise922.html.
4. Emma Childs and Harriet de Wit, "Regular Exercise Is Associated with Emotional Resilience to Acute Stress in Healthy Adults," *Frontiers in Physiology* 5 (2014): 161.
5. Abdullah Bora Ozkara et al., "The Role of Physical Activity in Psychological Resilience," *Baltic Journal of Sport and Health Sciences* 3, no. 102 (2016): 24–29.

6. Jasper A. J. Smits and Michael W. Otto, *Exercise for Mood and Anxiety Disorders: Therapist Guide* (New York: Oxford Univ. Press, 2010).

7. American Federation of Astrologers, "Astrology Correspondence Course [AFA SuperStar Course]," https://www.astrologers.com/learn-astrology/.

8. Editors, "Mars: Roman God," *Encyclopaedia Britannica* online, https://www.britannica.com/topic/Mars-Roman-god.

9. Edith Hamilton, *Mythology: Timeless Tales of Gods and Heroes* (New York: Black Dog & Leventhal, 2017).

10. Erskine P. Ausbrooks, Sandra P. Thomas, and Robert L. Williams, "Relationships Among Self-Efficacy, Optimism, Trait Anger, and Anger Expression," *Health Values* 19, no. 4 (1995): 46–54.

11. Howard Kassinove et al., "Self-Reported Anger Episodes in Russia and America," *Journal of Social Behavior and Personality* 12, no. 2 (1997): 301–24.

12. Sandra P. Thomas et al., "Anger and Cancer: An Analysis of the Linkages," *Cancer Nursing* 23, no. 5 (2000): 344–49.

13. LaVelle Hendricks et al., "The Effects of Anger on the Brain and Body," *National Forum Journal of Counseling and Addiction* 2, no. 1 (2013), http://www.nationalforum.com/Electronic%20Journal%20Volumes/Hendricks,%20LaVelle%20The%20Effects%20of%20Anger%20on%20the%20Brain%20and%20Body%20NFJCA%20V2%20N1%202013.pdf.

Chapter 11: Jupiter: Harbinger of Joy and Abundance

1. OWN, "Oprah on Making Things Happen in Your Life," Oprah.com, video, 1:01, http://www.oprah.com/own-digitaloriginals/oprah-on-making-things-happen-in-your-life-video.

2. Barbara L. Frederickson, "The Role of Positive Emotions in Positive Psychology: The Broaden-and-Build Theory of Positive Emotions," *American Psychologist* 56, no. 3 (2001): 218–26, https://www.ncbi.nlm.nih.gov/pmc/articles/PMC3122271/pdf/nihms-305177.pdf.

3. Barbara L. Fredrickson, "Gratitude, Like Other Positive Emotions, Broadens and Builds," from *The Psychology of Gratitude*, eds. Robert A. Emmons and Michael E. McCullough (New York: Oxford Univ. Press, 2004), 145–66, http://peplab.web.unc.edu/files/2018/11/fredrickson2004.pdf.

4. Susan Folkman and Judith Tedlie Moskowitz, "Positive Affect and the Other Side of Coping," *American Psychologist* 55, no. 6 (2000): 647–54, http://citeseerx.ist.psu.edu/viewdoc/download?doi=10.1.1.596.8982&rep=rep1&type=pdf; and Guido Veronese, Cindy Sousa, and Federica Cavazzoni, "Survival and Resilience Among Palestinian Women: A Qualitative Analysis Using Individual and Collective Life Events Calendars," *Violence Against Women*, May 4, 2020, published online ahead of print.

5. Karina A. de Allicon, "A Mindfulness Toolkit to Optimise Incident Management and Business Continuity Exercises," *Journal of Business Continuity and Emergency Planning* 13, no. 3 (2020): 220–29.

6. Shane Sinclair et al., "Sympathy, Empathy, and Compassion: A Grounded Theory Study of Palliative Care Patients' Understandings, Experiences, and Preferences," *Palliative Medicine* 31, no. 5 (2017): 437–47.

7. Folkman and Moskowitz, "Positive Affect and the Other Side of Coping," http://citeseerx.ist.psu.edu/viewdoc/download?doi=10.1.1.596.8982&rep=rep1&type=pdf.

8. Abraham M. Rutchick et al., "Future Self-Continuity Is Associated with Improved Health and Increases Exercise Behavior," *Journal of Experimental Psychology: Applied* 24, no. 1 (2018): 72–80, http://www.columbia.edu/~ms4992/Pubs/2018_Rutchick-Slepian-Reyes-Pleskus-Hershfield_JEPA.pdf.

Chapter 12: Saturn: Life Purpose and Discipline

1. TED-Ed, "How to Live to Be 100+ — Dan Buettner," YouTube video, 19:39, posted April 17, 2013, https://youtu.be/ff40YiMmVkU.

2. TED-Ed, "How to Live to Be 100+," https://youtu.be/ff40YiMmVkU.

3. Liz Greene, *Saturn: A New Look at an Old Devil* (San Francisco: Red Wheel/Weiser, 2011).

4. Ibid.

5. Aliya Alimujiang et al., "Association Between Life Purpose and Mortality Among US Adults Older Than 50 Years," *JAMA Network Open* 2, no. 5 (2019): e194270, https://jamanetwork.com/journals/jamanetworkopen/fullarticle/2734064?utm_source=For_The_Media&utm_medium=referral&utm_campaign=ftm_links&utm_term=052419.

6. Mara Gordon, "What's Your Purpose? Finding a Sense of Meaning in Life Is Linked to Health," *Shots*, NPR, May 25, 2019, https://www.npr.org/sections/health-shots/2019/05/25/726695968/whats-your-purpose-finding-a-sense-of-meaning-in-life-is-linked-to-health.

7. Stephanie A. Hooker and Kevin S. Masters, "Purpose in Life Is Associated with Physical Activity Measured by Accelerometer," *Journal of Health Psychology* 21, no. 6 (2016), https://journals.sagepub.com/doi/abs/10.1177/1359105314542822; and Eric S. Kim, Victor J. Strecher, and Carol D. Ryff, "Purpose in Life and Use of Preventive Health Care Services" *PNAS* 111, no. 46 (2014): 16331–36, https://www.pnas.org/content/111/46/16331.full.

8. Edward L. Deci and Richard M. Ryan, "Hedonia, Eudaimonia, and Well-Being: An Introduction," *Journal of Happiness Studies* 9 (2008): 1–11, http://www.preptheday.com/uploads/1/2/0/0/120050120/hedonia_eudaimonia_and_well-being.pdf.

9. Frank Martela and Michael F. Steger, "The Three Meanings of Meaning in Life: Distinguishing Coherence, Purpose, and Significance," *Journal of Positive Psychology* 11, no. 5 (2016): 531–45.

10. Greene, *Saturn.*

11. Chenkai Wu et al., "Association of Retirement Age with Mortality: A Population-Based Longitudinal Study Among Older Adults in the USA," *Journal of Epidemiology & Community Health* 70, no. 99 (2016): 917–23.

12. Greene, *Saturn.*

Chapter 13: Chiron: Why Your Wound Is Your Wisdom

1. Todd B. Kashdan and Jennifer Q. Kane, "Post-Traumatic Distress and the Presence of Post-Traumatic Growth and Meaning in Life: Experiential Avoidance as a Moderator," *Personality and Individual Differences* 50, no. 1 (2011): 84–89.

2. Martha Beck, "The Key to Healing Emotional Wounds," *O, The Oprah Magazine*, November 2013, http://www.oprah.com/inspiration/martha-beck-how-to-heal-emotional -wounds.

3. TEDx Talks, "The Space Between Self-Esteem and Self-Compassion: Kristin Neff at TEDxCentennialParkWomen," YouTube video, 19:00, posted February 6, 2013, https://youtu.be/IvtZBUSplr4.

4. Nitika Chopra, "Episode 6: From Post-Traumatic Stress to Post-Traumatic Growth with Jennifer Racioppi," February 3, 2019, *The Point of Pain*, podcast, 56:27, https:// nitikachopra.com/podcast/from-post-traumatic-stress-to-post-traumatic-growth -jennifer-racioppi/.

5. Demetra George, *Astrology and the Authentic Self: Integrating Traditional and Modern Astrology to Uncover the Essence of the Birth Chart* (Lake Worth, FL: Nicolas Hays, 2008).

6. Barbara Hand Clow, *Chiron: Rainbow Bridge Between the Inner and Outer Planets* (St. Paul: Llewellyn, 1999).

7. Brian Clark, "Brave New World—Forward into the Fifties," A Place in Space website, https://www.aplaceinspace.net/pages/brave-new-world-forward-fifties.

Chapter 14: Uranus: Authenticity and Breakthrough

1. NASA Science: Solar System Exploration, "Uranus: In Depth," last modified December 19, 2019, https://solarsystem.nasa.gov/planets/uranus/in-depth/.

2. Francesca Gino, Maryam Kouchaki, and Adam D. Galinsky, "The Moral Virtue of Authenticity: How Inauthenticity Produces Feelings of Immorality and Impurity," *Psychological Science* 26, no. 7 (2015): 983–96, https://www.hbs.edu/faculty/Publication %20Files/Moral%20Virtue_7caef67d-e4c7-4b38-88c7-b98da81826a5.pdf.

3. Abigail A. Mengers, "The Benefits of Being Yourself: An Examination of Authenticity, Uniqueness, and Well-Being," *Master of Applied Positive Psychology (MAPP) Capstone Projects* 63 (August 2014), https://repository.upenn.edu/cgi/viewcontent .cgi?article=1064&context=mapp_capstone.

4. Megan E. Gilster, "Comparing Neighborhood-Focused Activism and Volunteerism: Psychological Well-Being and Social Connectedness," *Journal of Community Psychol ogy* 40, no. 7 (2012): 769–84.

5. Elizabeth A. Emley, "Social Movements and Health: The Benefits of Being Involved" (master's thesis, Bowling Green State University, May 2017), https://etd.ohiolink .edu/!etd.send_file?accession=bgsu1490715716992475&disposition=inline.

6. Richard Tarnas, *Prometheus the Awakener: An Essay on the Archetypal Meaning of the Planet Uranus* (Woodstock, CT: Spring Publications, 1994).

Chapter 15: Neptune: Intuition and Spiritual Development

1. Marlynn Wei, "New Research on How Yoga Boosts Your Immune System," *Psychol ogy Today*, February 22, 2018, https://www.psychologytoday.com/us/blog/urban -survival/201802/new-research-how-yoga-boosts-your-immune-system.

2. Deepak Chopra, "How Meditation Helps Your Immune System Do Its Job," Chopra Center, January 14, 2015, https://chopra.com/articles/how-meditation-helps-your -immune-system-do-its-job.

3. Emma Seppälä, "The Surprising Health Benefits of Spirituality," *Psychology Today*, August 8, 2016, https://www.psychologytoday.com/us/blog/feeling-it/201608/the -surprising-health-benefits-spirituality; and Sedighe Forouhari et al., "Relationship Between Religious Orientation, Anxiety, and Depression Among College Students: A Systematic Review and Meta-Analysis," *Iranian Journal of Public Health* 48, no. 1 (2019): 43–52.

4. Gordon W. Allport and Michael J. Ross, "Personal Religious Orientation and Prejudice," *Journal of Personality and Social Psychology* 5, no. 4 (1967): 432–43.

5. David Spurgeon, "People Who Sleep for Seven Hours a Night Live Longest," *BMJ* 324, no. 7335 (2002): 446.

6. Jeffrey Kluger, "How to Wake Up to Your Creativity," *TIME*, April 30, 2017, https: //time.com/4737596/sleep-brain-creativity/.

7. Kluger, "How to Wake Up to Your Creativity," https://time.com/4737596/sleep -brain-creativity/.

8. National Institutes of Health, "Sleep Deprivation Increases Alzheimer's Protein," April 24, 2018, https://www.nih.gov/news-events/nih-research-matters/sleep-deprivation -increases-alzheimers-protein.

9. Nina E. Fultz et al., "Coupled Electrophysiological, Hemodynamic, and Cerebrospinal Fluid Oscillations in Human Sleep," *Science* 366, no. 6465 (2019): 628–31, https://science.sciencemag.org/content/366/6465/628.

10. Juliette Palisson et al., "Music Enhances Verbal Episodic Memory in Alzheimer's Disease," *Journal of Clinical and Experimental Neuropsychology* 37, no. 5 (2015): 503–17; Valorie N. Salimpoor et al., "Anatomically Distinct Dopamine Release During Anticipation and Experience of Peak Emotion to Music," *Nature Neuroscience* 14 (2011): 257–62; American College of Cardiology, "Music Boosts Exercise Time During Cardiac Stress Testing: Listening to Upbeat Music May Help Prolong Activity and Participation; Results May Have Broader Implications for Exercise in General," news release, *ScienceDaily*, March 1, 2018, https://www.sciencedaily.com/releases /2018/03/180301094811.htm; and Brian Wansink and Koert van Ittersum, "Fast Food Restaurant Lighting and Music Can Reduce Calorie Intake and Increase Satisfaction," *Psychological Reports* 111, no. 1 (2012): 228–32.

11. Bessel van der Kolk, *The Body Keeps the Score* (New York: Penguin, 2015).

Chapter 16: Pluto: Transformation and Transmutation

1. Robert Graves, *The Greek Myth: The Complete and Definitive Edition* (New York: Viking, 2018).

2. "Transmutation," Lexico.com, accessed July 18, 2020, https://www.lexico.com/definition /transmutation.

3. Jeff Green, *Pluto: The Evolutionary Journey of the Soul, Volume I* (St. Paul, MN: Llewellyn, 1985).

4. Pema Chödrön, *When Things Fall Apart: Heart Advice During Difficult Times* (Boston: Shambhala, 1997).

5. Neda Semnani, "A Harvard Psychologist Explains Why Forcing Positive Thinking Won't Make You Happy," *Washington Post*, September 23, 2016, https://www.washington

post.com/news/inspired-life/wp/2016/09/23/forcing-positive-thinking-wont-make -you-happy-says-this-harvard-psychologist/.

6. Joanne V. Wood, W. Q. Elaine Perunovic, and John W. Lee, "Positive Self-Statements: Power for Some, Peril for Others," *Psychological Science* 20, no. 7 (2009): 860–66; and June Yeung Chun and Vivian Miu Chi, "When Self-Help Materials Help: Examining the Effects of Self-Discrepancy and Modes of Delivery of Positive Self-Statements," *Journal of Positive Psychology* 11, no. 2 (2016): 163–72, https://commons.ln .edu.hk/cgi/viewcontent.cgi?article=3651&context=sw_master.

7. Ed Yong, "The Peril of Positive Thinking—Why Positive Messages Hurt People with Low Self-Esteem," *ScienceBlogs*, May 27, 2009, https://scienceblogs.com/notrocket science/2009/05/27/the-peril-of-positive-thinking-why-positive-messages-hurt.

8. Mark D. Alicke and Olesya Govorun, "The Better-Than-Average Effect," in *Studies in Self and Identity: The Self in Social Judgment*, eds. Mark D. Alicke, David. A. Dunning, and Joachim I. Kreuger (New York: Psychology Press, 2005).

9. Tali Sharot, "The Optimism Bias," TED2012, video, 17:25, February 2012, https: //www.ted.com/talks/tali_sharot_the_optimism_bias/.

10. Karen A. Baikie and Kay Wilhelm, "Emotional and Physical Health Benefits of Expressive Writing," *Advances in Psychiatric Treatment* 11, no. 5 (2005): 338–46, https://www.americansforthearts.org/sites/default/files/338full.pdf.

Conclusion

1. Madeline Miller, *Circe* (New York: Back Bay Books, 2020).

Index

Note: Italic page numbers refer to illustrations.

Index

About the Author

JENNIFER RACIOPPI is a transformational coach and professional astrologer. Her popular private practice often has a waiting list due to high demand. Several thousand people also work with Jennifer through her online Lunar Logic Moon School challenge, group programs, and live public-speaking classes. Her clients in these programs and her one-on-one practice have included creatives, celebrities, C-level corporate leaders, seven-figure entrepreneurs, and everyone in between. Jennifer is the resident astrology expert for Well+Good, where she's written a weekly column titled "Cosmic Health" since 2017. In the past, she served as the resident astrologer for Kate Northrup's membership site Origin and was a regular contributor to Reebok, *The Numinous*, and Netflix Family. Her work has also appeared in *Cosmopolitan*, American Eagle, and mindbodygreen. Prior to her career as a coach and astrologer, Jennifer received a degree in creative writing and climbed the corporate ladder as a top performer. After leaving the corporate world, she formally studied integrative wellness, positive psychology, and astrology. To learn more about Jennifer and her work, visit JenniferRacioppi.com.